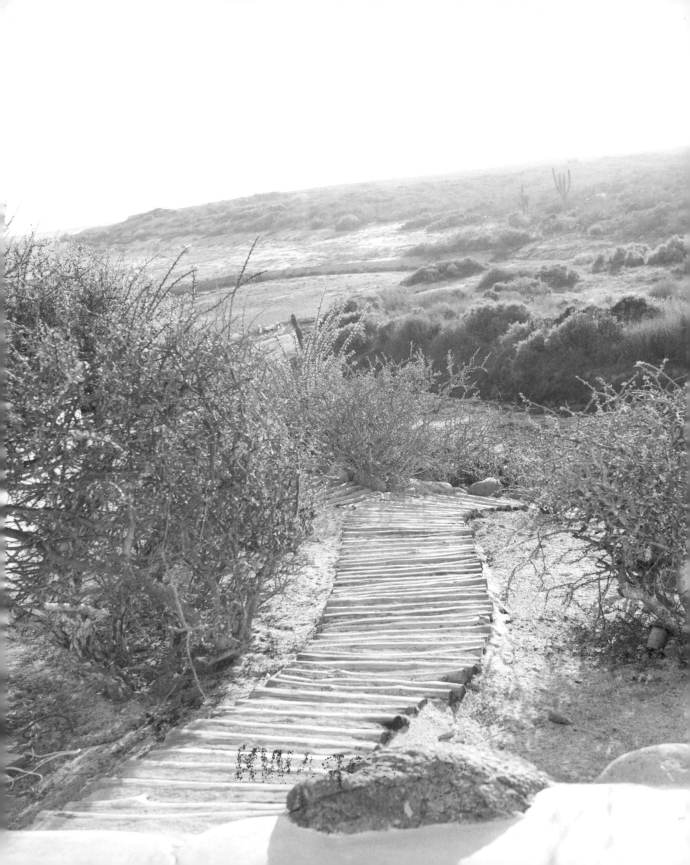

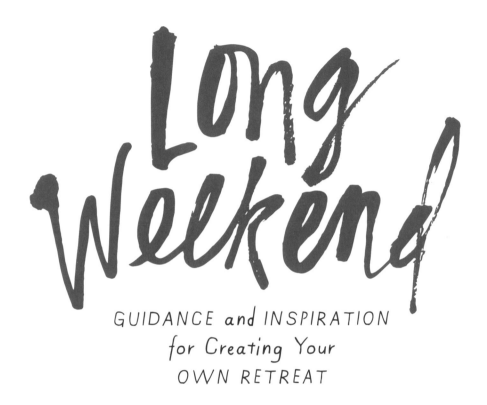

Long Weekend

GUIDANCE and INSPIRATION
for Creating Your
OWN RETREAT

RICHELLE DONIGAN and RACHEL NEUMANN
PHOTOGRAPHS by ERICKA McCONNELL

PARALLAX
PRESS

BERKELEY, CALIFORNIA

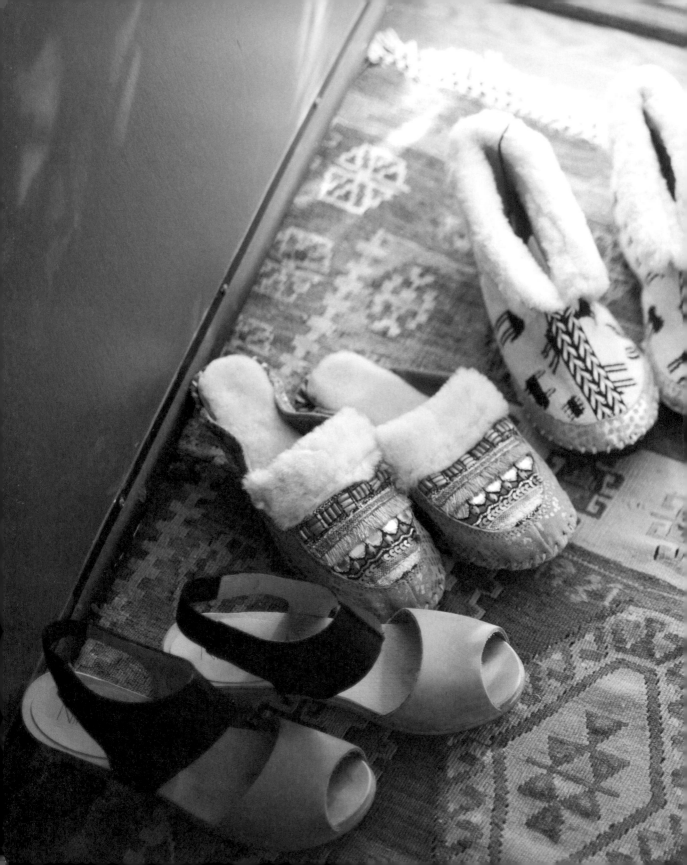

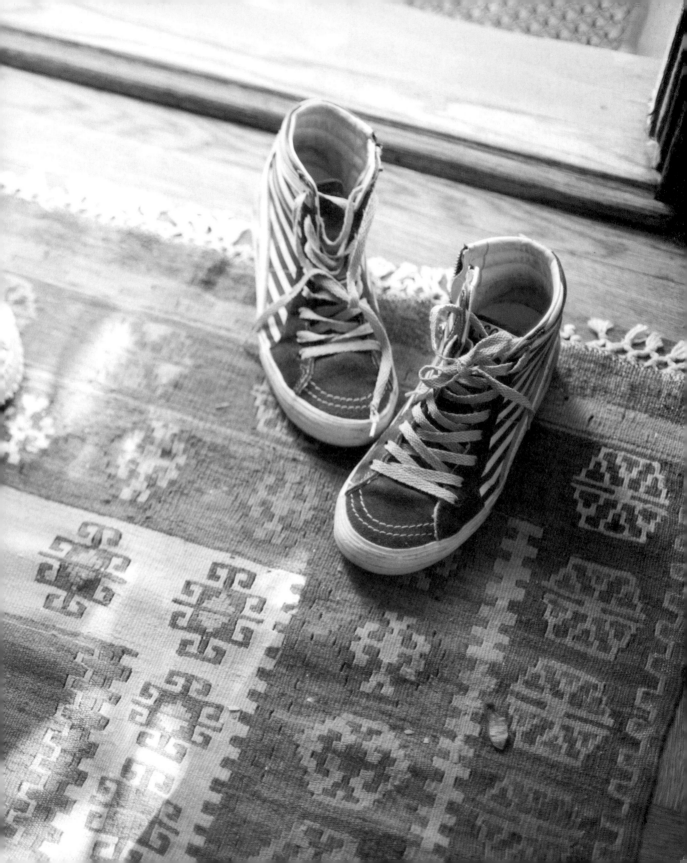

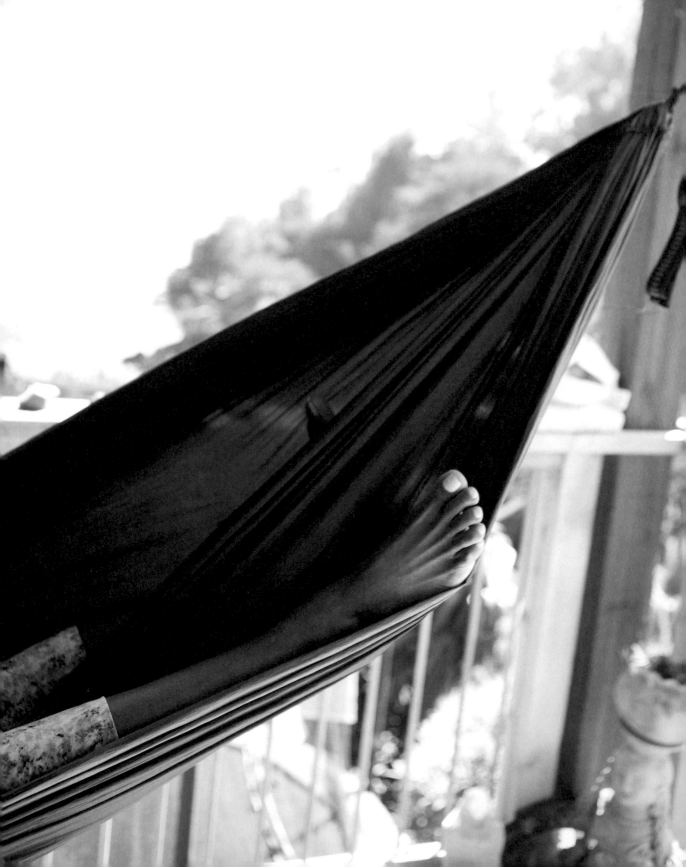

contents

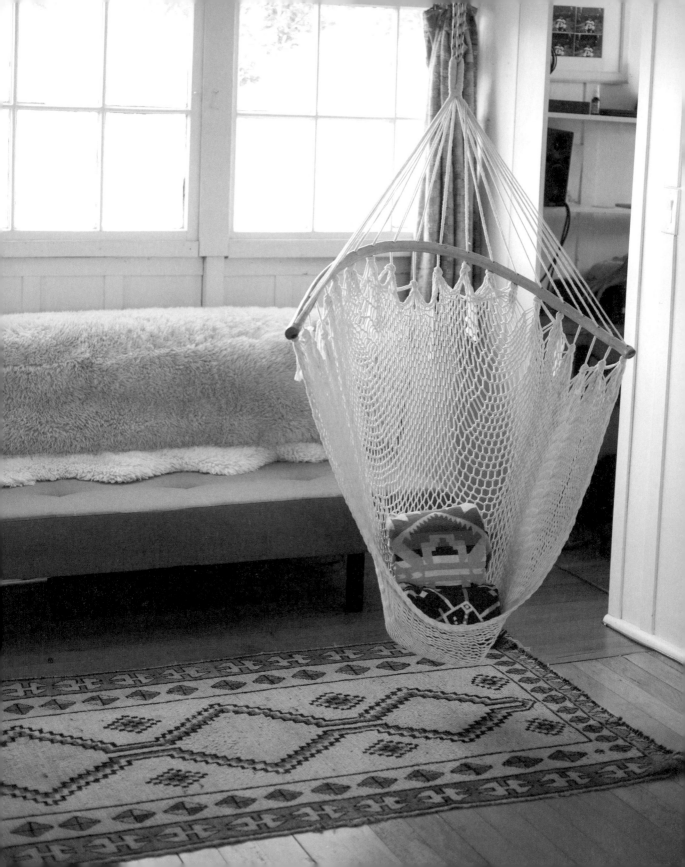

Introduction
What Is a Long Weekend?

When you think of a retreat, you may think of leaving home, traveling to some place beautiful, serene, and far away. How amazing it would be to leave it all behind for a few days and simply rest. But if and when we are able to "get away from it all," it can take a while to calm our busy minds. Our precious time away can become more about *doing* than *being*. We may find ourselves filling up the space with activity, anxiously checking work email or replaying stories in our heads. We may end up feeling the need for a retreat after our retreat!

Long Weekend is an invitation to *being*. We can be on retreat without going anywhere. It is an opportunity to create beautiful and serene moments right where we are—in our home, with ourselves, in our neighborhood or in nature, alone or with our family, friends, or community. We can also go away to be on retreat, but it's important that while traveling there, we don't get rushed or stressed. Taking our time is a radical and necessary act that gives us the opportunity to nurture the qualities inside that we also wish to cultivate in the world.

We offer ideas for each day of a three-day retreat, including activities that you can mix and match, as well as additional resources for meals, customizing your time, and ways to bring a little bit of the ease of a long weekend into your daily life.

A thousand-mile journey is begun with a single step.
—Lao Tzu

Our world is moving faster and faster. We can find ourselves depleted, overscheduled, and sleep-deprived, reaching for quick infusions of energy from endless cups of coffee or energy bars. This can float us for a while, until the inevitable crash that leads us back to dreaming, wishing, and planning our escape. *Long Weekend* will give you the tools to integrate and care for yourself in ways that support your daily well-being.

Taking time to go away and turn it all off—the phone, the TV, the computer, the "always on" way of life—positively recalibrates your whole body, your mind, and your senses. Maybe you have done a cleanse when you took out sugar, wheat, alcohol, or dairy and noticed that after a few days you were actually tasting your food. When you clear away the noise and busyness of the day-to-day, life gets sweeter. You can hear and feel the quiet, the subtleties of a moment. Your long weekend is a healing balm for the soul, a tonic for the spirit.

With all of the giving we do in a single day, we need to take time out to replenish and nourish ourselves. Taking a long weekend is about giving yourself time for simplicity and balance, an extended pause from the usual. With clear planning and deliberate intentions, we can recharge, refresh, and gain resilance to carry us forward for our work in the world.

Rain falls from the sky, the sun shines, then night falls. There is a rhythm, a cyclical nature to things, and most of us feel out of step. We may feel that we are behind the ball. We may feel like there are never enough hours in the day or days in the week. We can feel the "if onlys" adding up. We are tired, stretched. Maybe we are working with some dis-ease in the physical body that is taking its toll. In front of the

What a Long Weekend Is

Crafting time for yourself in the ways you find most restorative and nourishing

Time to drop into yourself and what matters to you

Creative time

Deep rest

Silent time

Space for joy

Nourishment

Being rather than doing

television may be the only place we are actually getting some time to ourselves. This feeling is one of being out of balance.

Listen to your longings. You are hearing the deepest part of yourself speaking to you. Take the time to ask, "What would you love?"

In these pages there are recipes and tools for fun, health, and wellness. Give yourself permission to be in your own flow while reading. What if creating ease were as simple as rolling over in your sleep? It can be. Imagine saying "Yes!" to a few days of doing only what you desire. Nothing to *be* but what you choose. No time frame, no deadlines, no schedule.

Imagine saying yes to sweet languishing, to stopping to look at the beauty that surrounds you whether you are in the city or in the country, near the ocean or in the mountains. There is beauty everywhere, if you look for it. What would it be like to walk around your block or neighborhood on the hunt for the exquisite in everything?

You might find yourself saying yes to taking the time to play games, to draw or color, to read, or to dance or sing along to all the songs you love at the top of your voice. What we look for and hold space for we will find.

This is a time to remember who you are and maybe add a few new grooves.

Come journey with us. Take a moment now and listen to your breathing. Come find your way.

— *Richelle and Rachel*

What a Long Weekend Is Not

Working from home

A family vacation

Fitting yourself into an already pre-packaged and impersonal schedule

A work trip

A full-on party weekend

A weekend of taking care of the errands on your to-do list

A weekend of taking care of others

Self-Care Is Taking Space for Ourselves and Each Other

Our true home, Zen Master Thich Nhat Hanh says, is available to us right here in the present moment. Our breath is our light, leading the way back to ourselves. Often, our mind is going one way and our bodies another. We sit at a computer, thinking of something that is coming in the future or that happened in the past. When we stop and bring our awareness to our breath and bring our mind back to our body, then we have arrived. We are home.

Many of us are always running. We go from here to there, putting out fires, fixing things, doing things, making things happen, trying to make things better. We feel we don't have time to stop. When we do have a moment, we may want to collapse, to not think, to distract ourselves from our own mind.

We can take space for ourselves and each other. To stop and breathe and feel and enjoy requires awareness, and awareness requires our intention. We are taught that our lives depend on doing and running and keeping on doing. But in reality they don't. Our lives, and this world, depend on us living more in harmony with ourselves and each other, in alignment with our true intention.

This book is for you. Even when you feel you don't have time to get away, that you can't leave work or family, this book will help you plan for a little breathing space. It's for the makers and the healers, the artists, the activists, the caretakers and the caregivers who cannot imagine finding time for a break and just want everything to pause, for a moment, so they can breathe.

What a Long Weekend Can Be

Alone

With good friends

With siblings

Celebratory

A time to mourn

Quiet

Simple

Silly

At home

At a friend's home

At a cabin or home that you rent

Camping

Take a day—one day that is not arriving or returning—for yourself. We offer inspiration and suggested itineraries. It is not a rulebook.

You don't need to spend a lot of money or go far away to retreat and refresh. A long weekend can take place at a friend's house, or even at your own home, if you have the discipline not to use that time for errands and clean up.

We encourage you to create your own retreat. A long weekend is an opportunity for self and group caretaking for the purpose of restoring yourself and your loved ones so that you can do the work that you need to do in the world. It is not about paying someone to take care of you for a moment but rather taking the time to take care of yourself, build your community, and feast on beauty and laughter.

Caring for myself is not self-indulgence, it is self-preservation, and that is an act of political warfare.
—Audre Lorde

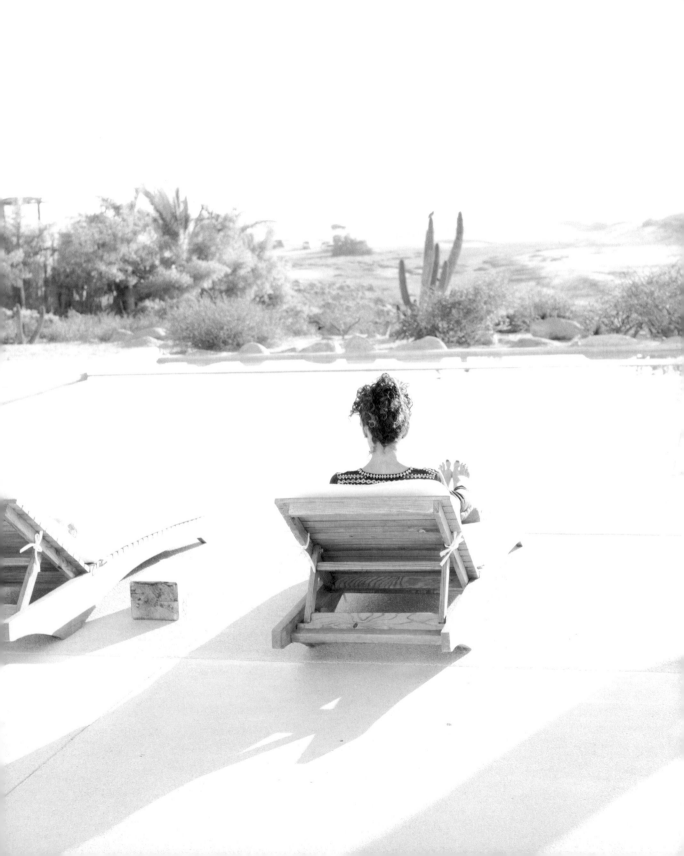

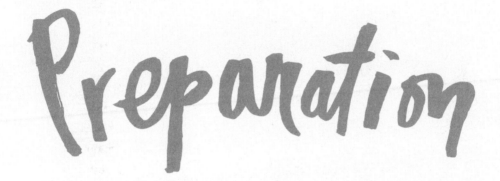

Preparation

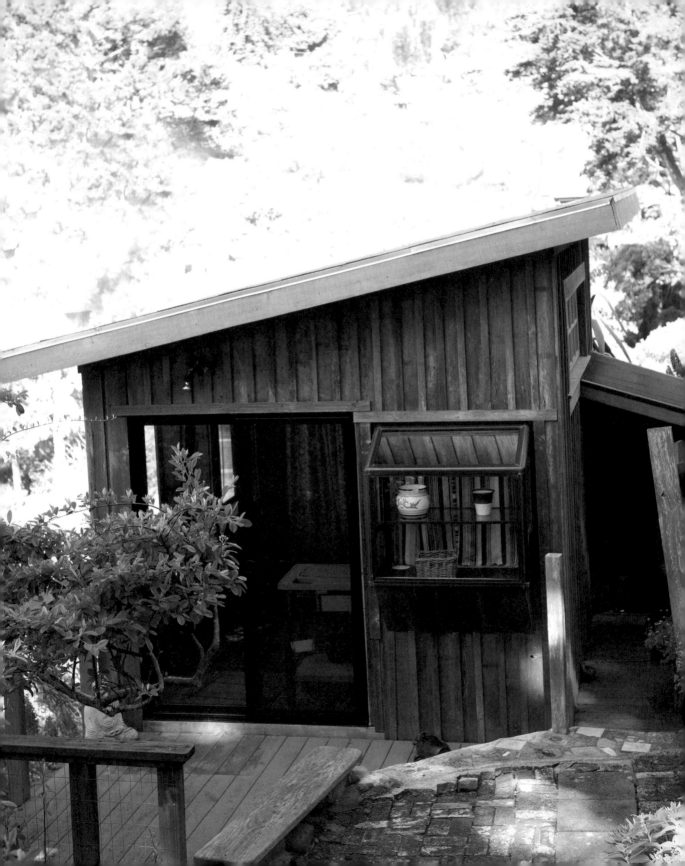

Deciding to Go on Retreat

There are times when we contemplate something we know would be good for us, playing with the idea of what we would love or how it may work, and we just keep playing with the idea, thinking about it, but never make a decision.

We keep it out there somewhere in *someday, when I have time* (or space), in the land of *wouldn't that be nice,* or *if only* . . . . It's a place we rarely find our way back to actualizing. The word *de-cide* literally means *to cut away.* So if you cut away the mental noise and being caught up in busy-ness, what would you need? Actions and resources are necessary, but the first step is committing to caring for yourself.

Is there a time when you made a decision that was so clear that you stuck to it and could not be moved? Remember what it felt like to make that decision. Allow that feeling to blossom and grow inside of you.

If you wish to advance in any sphere, the best way is to take a retreat.
–Pico Ayer

The most challenging part of a long weekend retreat is making the time to go and sticking to your plan.

Take a moment now and listen to your breathing. Follow your in-breath and your out-breath for three complete breath cycles.

You can do this.

Go ahead.

Now look at your calendar.

Imagine three days blocked out with your name and *Long Weekend* written across the top.

See it there.

Write it in.

You can figure out the rest later: where, with whom, what to do. The most important part is to make and save that time.

Mark your calendar in ink. It can be for the weekend coming up or for one that is months away. Then start telling people right away: your work, your family, your friends, and whoever needs to know.

Richelle:

I remember my journey with this. I wanted to go away and create some time that was just about me. I needed it; I was exhausted; it was time. But it stayed in my head as a dream, not a decision. I was great at creating retreats for others but I myself had not been on one in years. I had fooled myself into thinking that creating retreats and teaching at them was somehow the same as taking one. So I began to dream about going on retreat, alone.

Months went by, then a year came and went, then another, until I caught myself playing the someday game. I decided in that very moment to go on retreat for myself. I put down dates on my big old-school calendar. Of course things came up that wanted to pull me this way and that. Some really seemed more important, for a moment. "After all, I could go another weekend." "I could reschedule, couldn't I?" No! I had decided, for myself, that this was the most important thing on my schedule. I was the most important thing. I stopped the thoughts in their tracks. I redirected them so that they stayed in alignment with what I had decided. This was for my well-being. I kept my word. I went on those very dates. The place I went wasn't far from home; in fact, it was only about an hour away, and it was perfect.

The ocean, one room, my books, beautiful sleep, my pace, my time. It changed my life. I came back more myself. I had more to give and it was easier. One of the most important things that I had created was a place in me that knew this was an option. Now retreats are a regular occurrence for me. I take them with my partner, with others, or alone. It was so good for the whole of my life. It was as if layers of tiredness came off of everything. I was new.

Setting Your Intention

How you retreat, where you go, and who you go with will all be determined by your intention. You may want it all—time with loved ones, time alone, time in nature, time in the city, creative time, quiet time, exercising time, time to think about next steps or mark life transitions. You don't need to get it all in one weekend! There can be many long weekends, but they will be most satisfying if you are clear on what your priority is, how you want to use this time.

Take a few moments when you will not be interrupted and ask yourself what is most important to you in your three days away. Let yourself listen to whatever comes up, even if it seems selfish, wrong, or silly. Thoughts will come up that will counter the wishes that are arising; look at these thoughts with compassion and let them dissolve into the nothingness from which they came. There is no need for judgment or qualifiers. Breathe.

From this place of *choosing yourself*, again and again, begin to craft your intention for your weekend. What are your top three priorities? Rest? Being in nature? Long unhurried conversations? Connecting with yourself in quiet so that you can actually hear yourself and know more clearly what you would *love* to be doing? The intention you create will be your inner road map, a guide that will support you in creating the retreat that will most powerfully serve you.

Another world is not only possible, she is on her way.
—Arundhati Roy

Take up a pen and a piece of paper. At the top of the
page write:

What would I love?

Now look inward. Allow yourself to be introspective. Let the
writing unfold over a few days or a week.

Don't censor yourself.

Feel free to contradict yourself, to write down what feels
huge and impossible.

Now take a moment to breathe in. Breathe in your
worthiness and exhale your judgments and doubts. Let
them go.

You may want to say to yourself,

Breathing in, I am love
Breathing out, I choose love

Repeat this often.

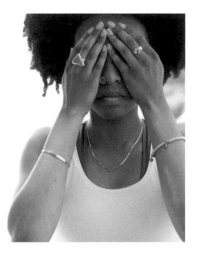

Who's In?

Your intention will guide you to know if it is time to be alone or be on a journey with a crew.

If you have a small squad that you know nourishes you, by all means go away together. Just keep it small. As your group grows, logistics get exponentially more complicated. You will need to think differently about a space that will fit all of you, your food, sleeping space, and activities. It will be important to be clear on the plan, as people have different needs and expectations. That said, being away with other people who inspire and nurture you may be exactly what you need. You can also support each other, motivate each other, and listen to each other in a way that only happens when a group gets together with time and space to breathe and be.

If you do go with other people, make sure to be transparent and to have clear communication in advance on the issues that can get trickiest: money, food, tasks, and needs (concerning noise, allergies, and the like). Before you invite people, think about what you will and won't compromise on and which people are easy for you to talk to and be with.

The real question is, what would *you* love? What will best fit your intention? If you choose to retreat with one or more loved ones, it helps to get crystal clear about what that time will look like and feel like, including the time and the organizing that lead up to your long weekend. Keep referring to your intention, your inner road

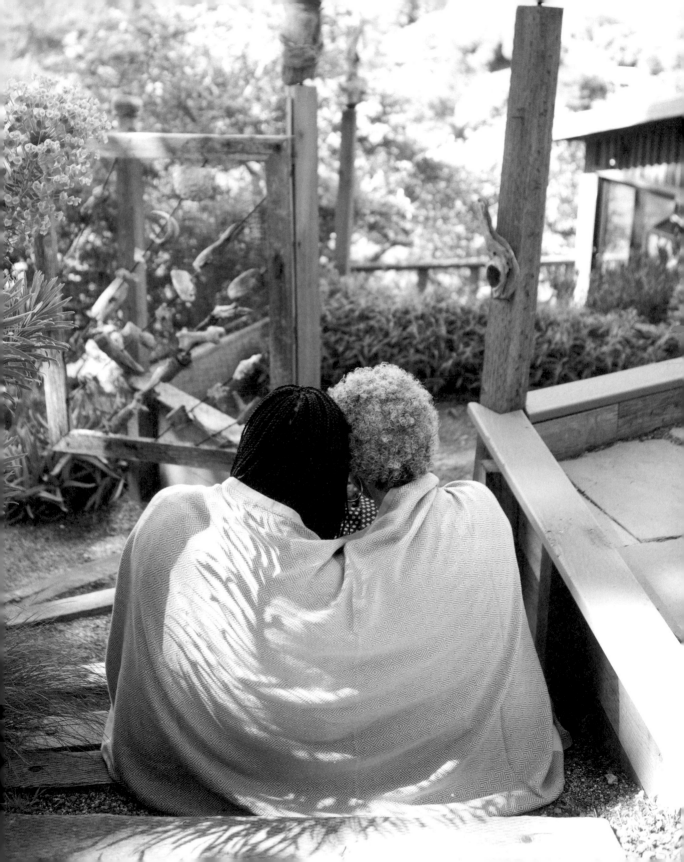

map, so that you know when you are veering off course. Encourage whomever you have chosen to accompany you to create an intention for themselves and to share it with you; likewise you can share yours with them.

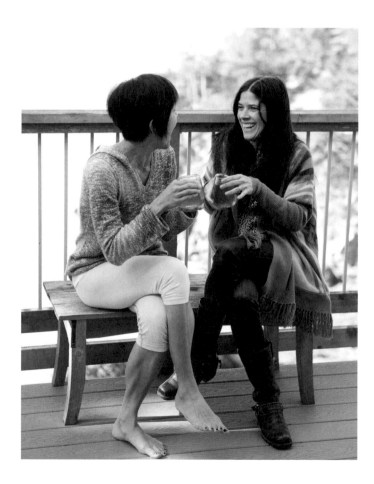

Courageous Conversations

Being with other people can be relaxing and nourishing, and it is even more so when you can be courageous about sharing your needs and concerns in advance. If you are doing any of the organizing and are inviting the other people, state your intention in the invitation so people can be clear from the beginning what they're getting into and what it will be like. And ask if they have intentions to share. *It's fine not to compromise on your intention. Just make sure you communicate it!*

There must be those among whom we can sit down and weep and still be counted as warriors.
—Adrienne Rich

Some questions to ask yourself and your group before planning begins:

o What are each person's goals and intentions for the weekend?

o How far away can you go?

o Do you want to be in town or in nature?

o How much money can you spend, if any?

o Do you want to split up the cooking or not cook at all?

o How much privacy do you need?

o What agreements on activities do you want to make in advance? Will you send out an agenda?

o Is there anything that is non-negotiable? Quiet hours, food allergies, or other needs?

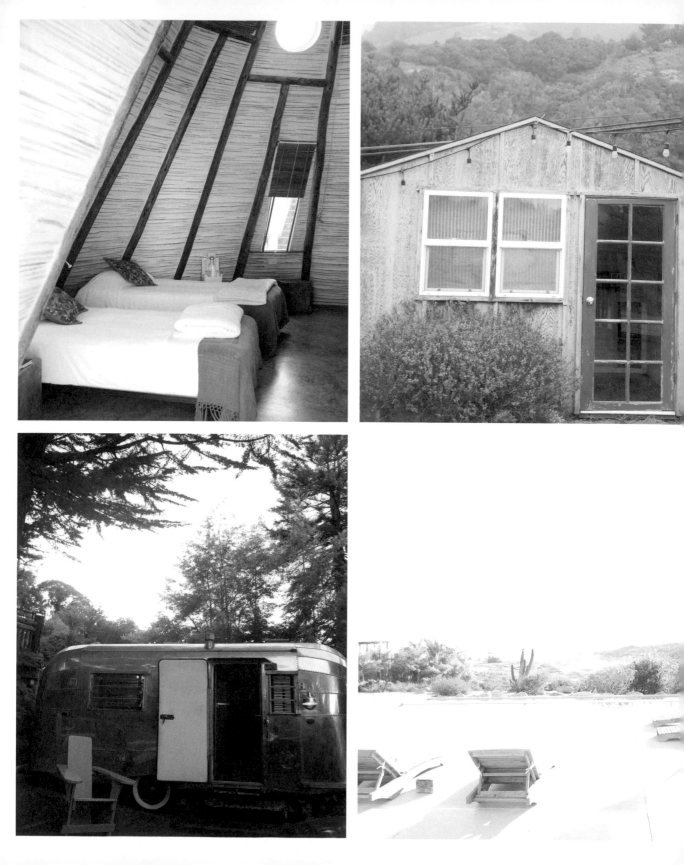

Where Are You Going?

If you are alone, consider whether you like traveling alone and how you like to travel. The bus, car, train, or plane can all be part of your journey. If you don't like driving, don't go somewhere a few hours away unless you have a designated driver or a good public transit route. If you are alone, make sure you are traveling to a place where you feel safe. If you are traveling with a small group, be aware of how much cost and effort it will take each person to participate.

Here are some potential destinations you might consider:

Your Own Home
If you can switch off your phone, not do household chores, and dedicate yourself to your retreat, the place where you live can become your personal sanctuary for a long weekend.

A Friend's Home
You don't have to wait until you can head far away to enjoy a long weekend. For time away from the day-to-day, a friend's house can be as relaxing as a faraway spot and requires far less planning.

A Retreat Center
Many contemplative traditions offer a place to stay for quiet reflection, writing, and personal inquiry. If you research nearby retreat centers, you may be surprised by the resources in your area.

Near Water
Go to the nearest pond, lake, river, or ocean. Consider staying someplace nearby that has a pool, a hot tub, or a really good bathtub.

Mountains and Woods
Camping, or renting a cabin or recreational vehicle, can be easy ways to enjoy the mountains. Perhaps there is a kind of forest or tree that speaks to you. There is a quietness to trees that helps us become peaceful.

What is that magical place for you? Is it hunkering down in your own house and falling in love with your city again (or for the first time)? Is it walking on the beach with no destination or time frame to follow, letting the wind and the waves tell you their secrets? What would you *love*?

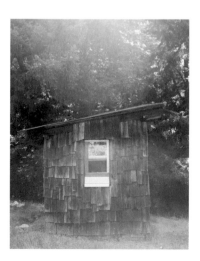

Preparing to Go

Have all of the conversations that you need to have well in advance so that you are able to completely let go once your long weekend begins.

Three to six months before you go
Set your intention and, with that as your guide, figure out where you are going. Reserve the space. Invite the people you most want to be with.

Three months before you go

o   Let people know you're going.

o   Get the time off from work.

o   Arrange childcare or petcare, if you need to.

o   Make it clear to people that you won't be reachable that weekend.

o   Start your packing list.

The month before you go

o   Make sure meals are arranged with your travel
    companions, if you have them. Set up agreements in
    advance about your time together, such as:

o   Will there be set times that are quiet?

o   How will meals be handled? Is one person in charge?
    Will you cook, eat out, order in? Make sure any costs
    are clear up front, so no one is expected to pay for
    anything she wasn't prepared to.

o   If you are retreating alone, still decide in advance
    how you would like to handle meals and whether you
    will be completely off-the-grid or if you will set aside
    time for checking in on phone/email etc. Make sure, if
    you are going someplace where you will be tempted
    to be online, that you decide in advance how you
    want to use or limit that time.

o   Write up your packing list. Review your intention.

o   Are you creating the best conditions you can to help
    that intention manifest?

The week before you go

o   Put your autoresponder on your email.

o   Change your voicemail message if you have one.

o   Pack early enough that there is time to add the things you forgot or take out things you won't need.

o   Check in with the crew that is coming with you, if any, and make sure everyone has all the information, including grocery and packing lists, driving information, and a write-up of any pre-arranged agreements about meals or schedule.

The day before you go

o   Check in with your intention. What would comprise a successful retreat?

o   Think about what you will return to. Consider cleaning your space before you go or leaving something beautiful to greet you on your return.

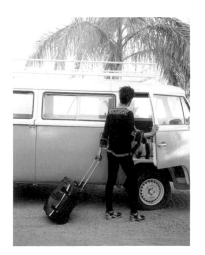

Packing List for a Long Weekend

_ A *schmatta*. "Schmatta" is a Yiddish word for a thin piece of cloth. It could be a sarong or some other kind of wrap that serves multiple purposes—as a quick drying towel, a place to sit, a scarf, an extra blanket, a skirt, a dress, a head wrap, whatever you need.

_ Thermos

_ Water bottle

_ Journal

_ Travel candle

_ What helps you sleep: eye pillow, headphones, earplugs

_ Books

_ Your favorite pillow

_ Musical instruments if you play

_ Playlists and something to play your music on

_ Favorite teas and coffees

_ Your most comfortable clothes, including something you enjoy sleeping in

_ A robe

_ A bathing suit

_ Yoga mat/props if you use them

_ Running shoes and/or other comfortable walking shoes

_ Sage

_ Lavender

_ Essential oils for bath or massage

_ Favorite lotions and potions (face oil, hair conditioner, perhaps the face mask you've been meaning to try)

_ Supplies for any projects you are working on during the weekend. This could be art supplies, face mask- or lotion-making ingredients, big rolls of butcher paper if people are going to be brainstorming together, collage materials, whatever you might need. (Each idea and activity in *Long Weekend* lists the supplies needed.)

_ A bell or timer for meditation

_ Bedside or altar offerings (such as a photograph, a book, a rock)

Packing

Regardless of whether you are staying at home or traveling to an alternate location, there are things you'll need to have with you. Pack them up. Having what you need close at hand will help you truly retreat. At the same time, consider packing light. Part of a retreat is the practice of being okay with what you have with you; you may have forgotten something you like for comfort. Before rushing back or buying it again, you might see what it's like to be without it.

Food

o   Depending on where you are traveling to and who your traveling companions are, you will either need to bring groceries or just bring snacks. Even if someone else is providing the food, bring snacks along. See our ideas in the Resources section at the back of the book for three days of simple, delicious meals.

o   You don't need to cook if you don't enjoy cooking. You can get pre-made food or have food delivered (depending on where you are staying).

o   If possible, find ways during these three days to make eating a practice and part of your retreat, whether you're alone or with others, rather than eating out. There are also many places that deliver wholesome meals right to the door.

o   If cooking is delightful to you and something you would love to do on your own or as a shared experience with others, make sure your kitchen is stocked with all you'll need.

o   Make your grocery list and do your shopping before your weekend. Include treats. See the food shopping list and Recipes in the Resources section for ideas.

Clothing

o   Bring clothes that will support whatever adventure you've chosen to have, whether it's walking on the beach, in the woods, in your yard, around the block, hiking; swimming; or yoga on the deck or in your den. Or maybe you'll choose to be in your favorite comfy clothes all weekend.

o   Bring something to keep warm.

o   If you are retreating with others, perhaps have everyone bring one silly or fancy item of clothing for a dinner together. Just because you are retreating doesn't mean you can't dress up if you enjoy it.

Books

o   Bring books that inspire, that book that you have been trying to read forever, or one that you just want to check out.

o   Bring a journal in which to record your experiences or draw.

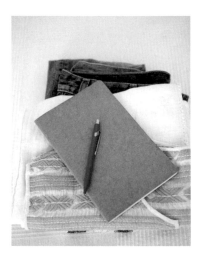

Art Supplies

o Bring basic art supplies with you for making a vision board and sketching. This could include: a blank book for sketching, a favorite pen and pencil, watercolors and brushes, scissors, and a glue stick. Consider bringing some old magazines to cut up or, if you don't have any, bring one you'd like to read and can cut up afterward.

Music

o Bring your music and perhaps get your playlist together, creating a soundtrack for your long weekend. Make sure you bring something you love to dance to. See the Playlists for a Long Weekend in the Resources section.

Altar

o Consider bringing sage to clear the air wherever you go. You may like to bring some other smell or herb that helps you feel at home. Is there something that as soon as you smell it your eyes close and your shoulders relax and you breathe deep and easy? Rose geranium, lavender, and cedar are all powerful options. Think about having an essential oil or dried sage that you can put in your pillow that will support your feeling of ease and rest. You may also choose to bring some things to create a small altar so that if you are away from home, there are things that ground you. This could include a photo, a candle, a shell, a rock, or anything else that centers you when you look upon it.

Consider *Not* Bringing

Your phone

Your computer

A camera (decide in advance, and with the group if you have one, whether you want to photograph the weekend or keep it private)

Hair dryer

Alcohol/drugs

Newspapers or magazines

Packing

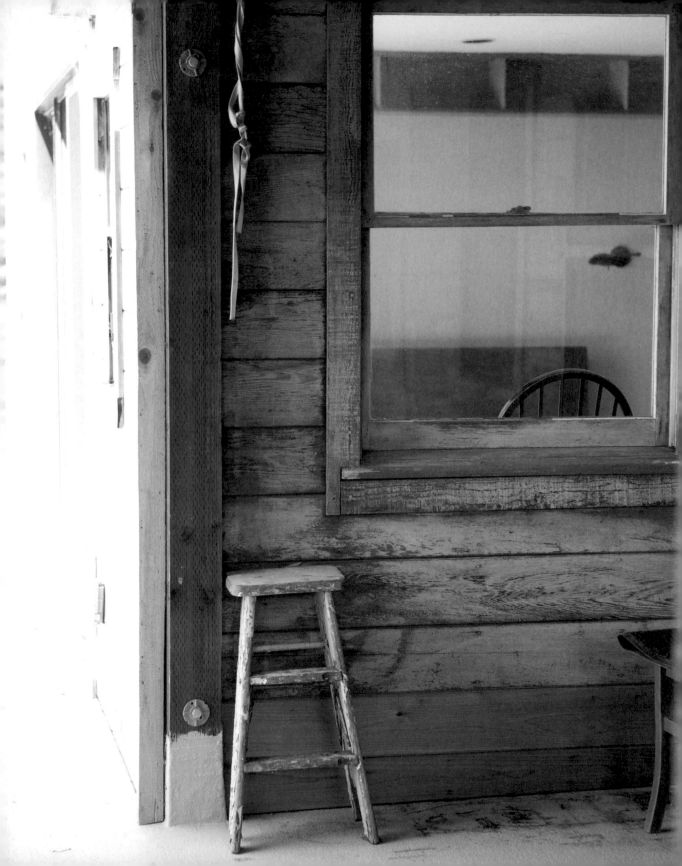

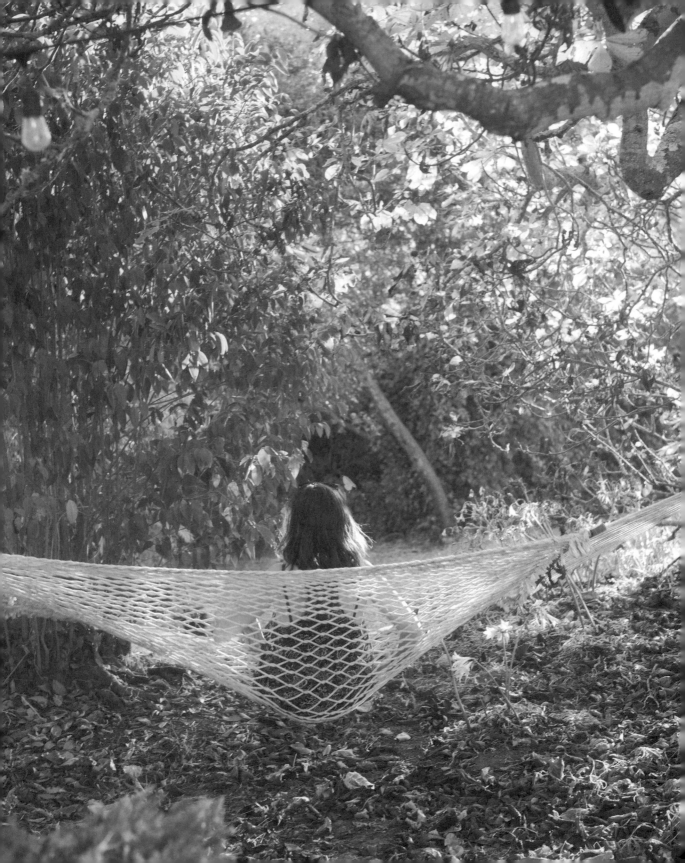

The Journey

Arrival

Gathering and Sitting Meditation

Setting Up Your Space

Practices for Grounding and Centering

Eating Meditation

Play

Ritual Bath

Deep Rest and Relaxation

DAY 1

Getting to Know Yourself
Outside of the Day-to-Day

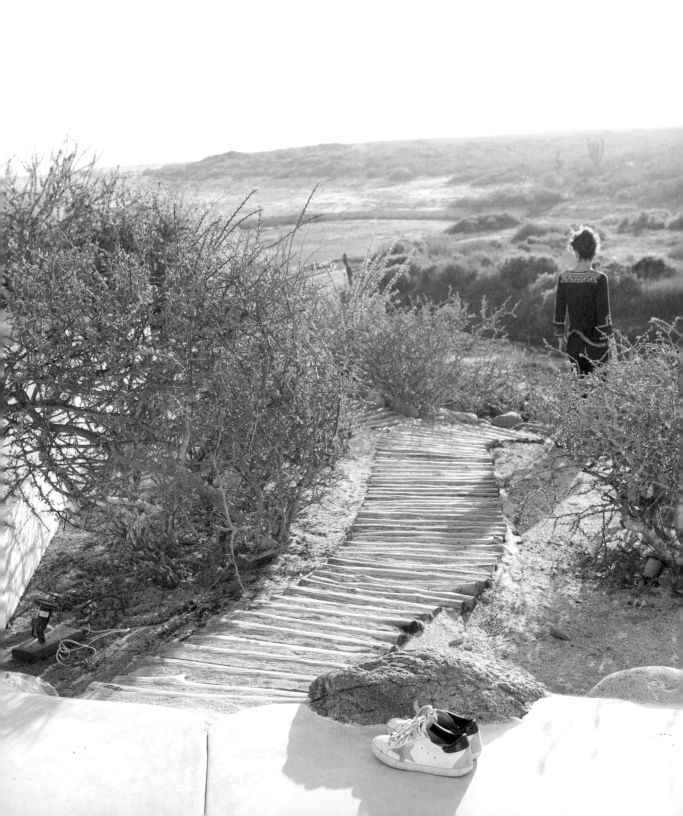

The Journey

Your first day really starts when you leave your day-to-day life and travel to your long weekend. Perhaps you are just going across town to a friend's house, or perhaps you are traveling hours or a day away by bus, train, car, or plane. Maybe you are staying at home, and just walking back into your house is your journey. Either way, mark that the time is different. Your Long Weekend begins now.

You may be tempted, as you pull away from your daily routine, to get a few more things done—a few last phone calls or texts or to-dos. You may experience a pull toward doing, to being on a schedule of some kind, to reading the news, or talking about or listening to things that cause the body to contract, or to things that just plain stress you out. You may find yourself thinking more about what you are not doing and missing out on while you are "away" from your daily life rather than experiencing that you are already in a different moment. But your long weekend has begun with the journey to where you will have your retreat.

It may be easier to catch your wandering thoughts if you have already imagined the night before how your day will be and have slept with your intention in mind. Then you can more easily redirect your thoughts and actions. The journey is the time to begin to unravel the pull to the familiar.

Your long weekend is a space to practice shifting ingrained habits. What is your body asking for? Day One is the time to listen to it.

To be fully alive, fully human, and completely awake is to be continually thrown out of the nest.
—Pema Chödrön

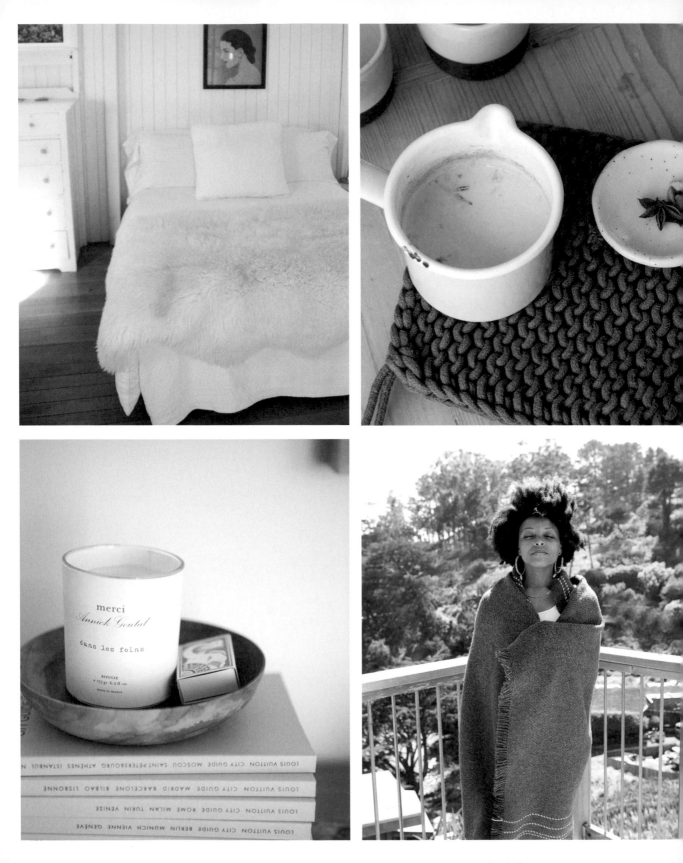

Arrival

Take time to arrive before unpacking or settling in.

Take your shoes off.

Walk around.

Say hello to your home for this long weekend.

Sit down.

Close your eyes.

Breathe.

You made it.

You have arrived.

Breathing in, I have arrived.
Breathing out, I am home.
—Thich Nhat Hanh

TRULY ARRIVING

As soon as you arrive, before you have even unpacked, take a moment to settle in.

Standing or seated, feel your feet on the floor. Take three deep breaths, breathing in long and breathing out slow. With each exhale, feel yourself more present in the space. Connect with what supports you, the structure that surrounds you, the earth beneath you.

With each inhale expand, take up more space; with each exhale root, drop down deeper. Not replacing one with the other. Do both, equally. Expand and root. Find yourself here. Grounded and expansive. Bring to your mind and heart your intention for your long weekend. Remember who you are *being*. There is a difference between getting rest and *being* rested. Bring to mind your intention. Embody it by taking another deep breath, expanding your intention from the center of your being outward until it fills the whole space and beyond.

Remember some of the words and the feelings of your intention and imagine playfully dropping them onto the floor. See the words written on the glass window pane: *rest, fun, ease, play*. See them written across the the ceiling, floating in the sky above. Now your intention for your weekend is woven into and through everything. If you begin to forget or move away from your intention, you'll be reminded, you'll see it in the window or as a cloud floats by, or you'll see it as the words scattered on the floor.

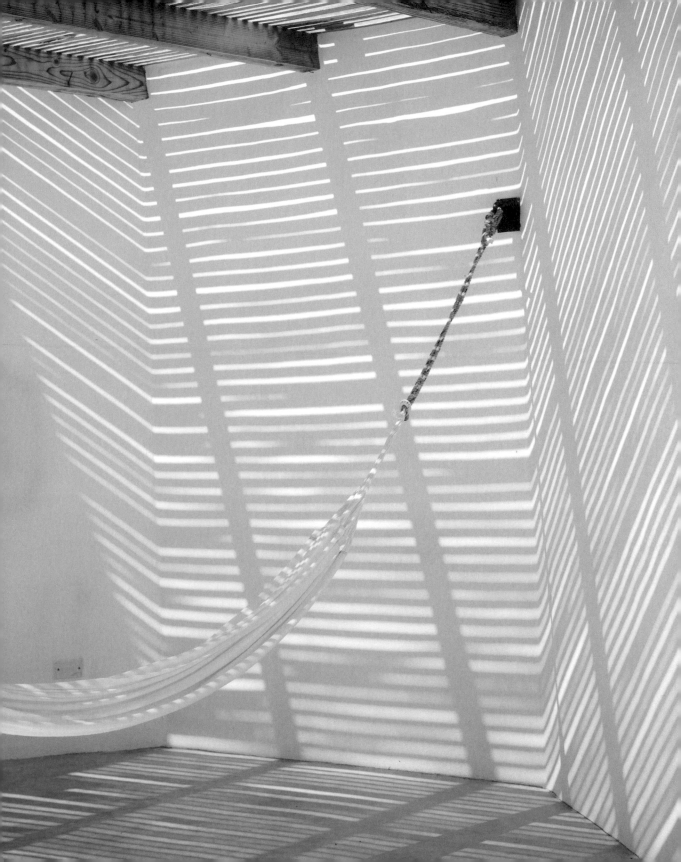

Gathering and Sitting Meditation

Meditation is simply the practice of focused paying attention, uniting breath and awareness. There are as many ways to meditate as there are waves in the ocean. It does not require any specific set of skills, beliefs, or body type. Meditation can be done while sitting or walking, chanting or in silence. There is even cooking, dancing, and eating meditation. Meditation is the training, the practice, of mindfulness, so that you can bring that mindful awareness into everything you do.

Zen Master Thich Nhat Hanh defines mindfulness as "the practice of being fully present and alive, body and mind united. Mindfulness is the energy that helps us to know what is going on in the present moment." Like most things, it gets easier with practice.

A sitting meditation can help ensure that your retreat starts off right. You may feel at first that you're not "doing" anything, especially when there is unpacking to be done and socializing and retreating to happen. Within minutes of arriving, you are grounding yourself in your body and breath and returning to your intention.

It is very common to feel with meditation that you are not doing it right or that it's "wasting your time." We can stare at a screen for hours but as soon as we choose five or ten minutes to meditate or pay attention, we can feel anxious or that we can't possibly wait for those few minutes to be over. Don't worry about doing it right. The doing, the sitting, is enough.

I learned to make my mind large, as the universe is large, so that there is room for contradictions.
—Maxine Hong Kingston

At every moment in meditation, you can choose to return to your breath. The choice to return to center over and over again—that is meditation. You can have thoughts without thoughts having you.

For arrival, we suggest a short sitting meditation. Here are two choices of meditations to try. One is Thich Nhat Hanh's instructions for how to sit. The other is a ten-minute guided meditation. If you do the guided meditation, consider reading it before you sit or, if you are in a group, having one person read it as the others sit.

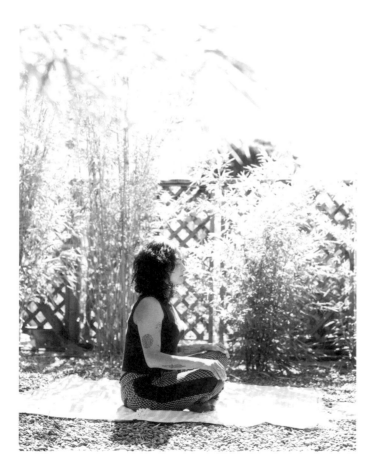

HOW TO SIT *by* THICH NHAT HANH

Sitting meditation should be a joy. Sit in such a way that you feel happy and relaxed for the entire length of the sitting. Sitting is not hard labor. It's an opportunity to enjoy your own presence, the presence of others, the earth, the sky, and the cosmos. There's no effort.

If you sit on a cushion, be sure it's the right thickness to support you. You can sit in the full- or half-lotus position, in a simple cross-legged position, or however you feel most comfortable. Keep your back straight and your hands folded gently in your lap. If you sit in a chair, be sure your feet are flat on the floor or on a cushion.

If your legs or feet fall asleep or begin to hurt during the sitting, just adjust your position mindfully. You can maintain your concentration by following your breathing and slowly and attentively changing your posture.

Allow all the muscles in your body to relax. Don't fight or struggle.

While sitting, begin by following your in-breath and out-breath. Whenever a feeling comes up, recognize it. Whenever a thought arises, identify it and recognize it. You can learn a lot from observing what's going on in your body and mind during the sitting meditation.

Most of all, sitting is a chance for you to do nothing. You have nothing at all to do; just enjoy sitting and breathing in and out. You can say to yourself as you sit:

Breathing in, I know I'm alive.
Breathing out, I smile to life, in me and around me.

Since you're breathing in and out, you know that you're alive. That's something worth celebrating. Sitting meditation is a way to celebrate life with your in-breath and your out-breath.

You may also say:
Breathing in, I have arrived.
Breathing out, I feel at home.

You don't need to run anymore. Your true home is in the here and the now. You are solid and free.

Enjoy the breathing in, the breathing out. Give up any struggle and enjoy sitting and smiling.

This is a privileged moment, having the opportunity to sit quietly like this. You are your own island. Nobody at this moment can ask you to do anything. Nobody will disturb you, no one has the right to ask you a question, or to ask you to go and wash the pots or clean the bathroom. This is your precious opportunity to relax and be yourself.

GUIDED SITTING MEDITATION

Find your way to your seat, noticing your steps along the way. Sit comfortably. As you sit, notice that you are supported. Notice there is that which is beneath you that is supporting you, whether it is a cushion, a chair, the floor, or a mat. There is support there.

You can close your eyes or just relax them by softening your gaze and letting it fall slightly downward.

Take a deep breath in and a long breath out. Do this a few times, just watching and experiencing your body as it expands and contracts with your breath. With each inhalation, allow for spaciousness and openness. With each exhalation, root down a little deeper into your foundation and what supports you. Just notice your breath. Again and again, bring your awareness back to your breath.

There will be thoughts that will come and go. Learn to let them go so the mind can be more spacious. So imagine that they are clouds, these thoughts. Imagine that there is a gentle wind that is moving them along. Keep gently bringing your attention back to your breath.

Bring full awareness to your breath, regarding it with curiosity. Noticing where it fills up first or where the last part of your exhaled breath comes from. Noticing its journey and pathway. The quality. The rhythm. The sound.

Your breath. Allow it to move throughout your body. You can begin to direct your out-breath to different parts of the body, to help release tension. You might start with your shoulders. If there is any tension there, allow that tension to drop down and be expelled with your breath.

If there is any tension in the neck or the legs or the feet, use your breath to bring relaxation to those places, focusing on one part of the body at a time. Use your breath to create spaciousness and ease. Each breath brings you deeper into yourself. Deeper into this moment. Let go of everything else.

Take a deep breath in. Breathe a long breath out. Deep breath in. Long breath out. Once again, inhale. And exhale. Gently bring your awareness back to your surroundings, very slowly opening and refocusing your eyes.

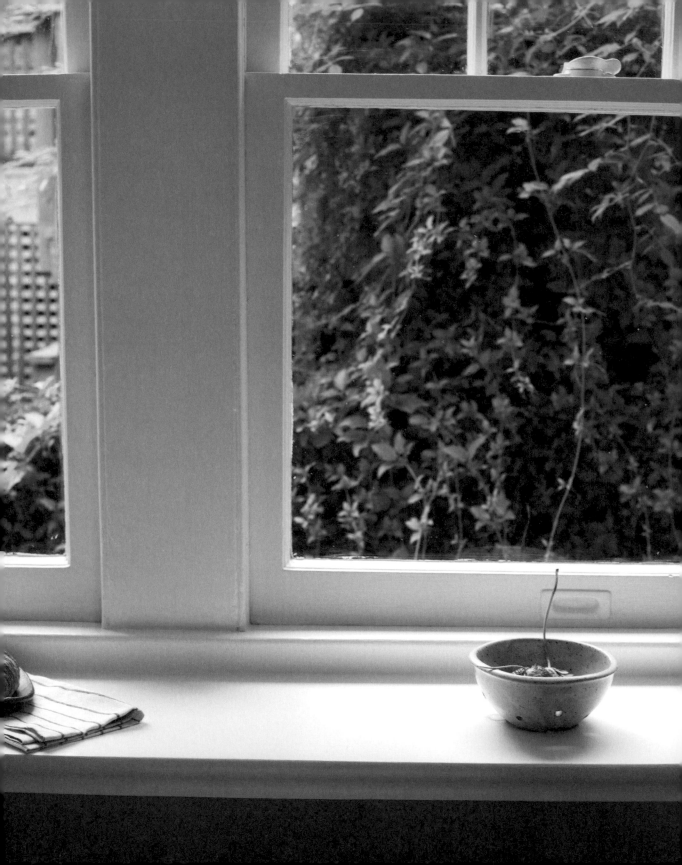

Setting up Your Space

Setting up your space may be as simple as putting on the teapot, some lovely music, your comfy clothes, and plopping in a chair with a book. Whatever it is, wherever it is, know that the retreat is happening now.

Do everything with ease, with awareness of your breath, and at your own pace. Place things where they are easy to see and access.

Set up the kitchen so food prep and meals are easy and fun.

Spritz one of your essential oils that you love and open the windows and let the air sweep out any stale energy.

Take up space. Reach your arms out, stand tall, and walk around your space, feeling your way to make it feel like home.

Clear your space with white sage, lavender or cedar

Take a small bundle (about the size of your thumb to forefinger circle) of dried sage, lavender or cedar.

Tie it together with string at both ends.

Light one of the ends with a match or lighter. The bundle should be smoking, not flaming.

Walk around the space, holding the bundle at arm's length and dispersing the smoke with your other hand.

Be very careful and, after clearing the space, ensure the fire is all the way out and there is no smoke before putting the bundle down.

SAVASANA

Savasana is Sanskrit for corpse pose, or the little death. It is
a profound practice of letting go of all that has come before.
The deepest version of this is to imagine letting go of your
body and residing wholly in the light of your being. In yoga
they say this is the hardest asana of all. So begin easy. Start
with letting go of everything that came before the moment
you are in. Listen to your breath, knowing that when you
do so you are present. We cannot breathe in the past, nor
can we take a breath in the future, so when we bring our
awareness to our breath, we are in the present. We have
truly arrived.

Practices for Grounding and Centering

Stretching and moving your body is key on this first day. As body and mind are two sides of the same phenomenon, when you move your body, you expand and shift your mindset.

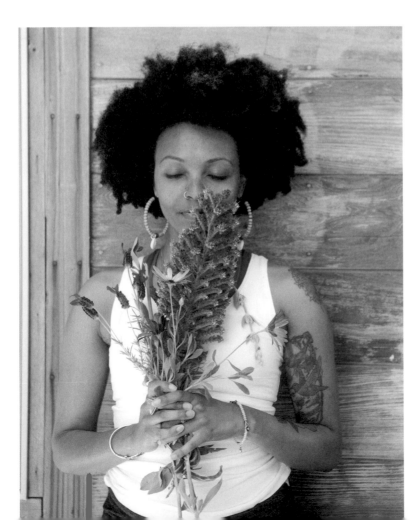

EARTH AND SKY

You can do this practice standing or seated.

Bring your awareness to your breath. Intentionally draw in a deeper breath and let it out really slow. As you exhale, draw your belly in slightly as you direct the breath all the way down your body through your feet into the earth.

Keeping that connection, inhale, and with your breath draw the energy up from the earth all the way up into your chest, expanding your heart space, and when you exhale, make it long and follow it as it moves all the way down your arms and out through your fingers.

Again, breathe in deeply, drawing the energy and breath up from the fingers, up the arms and arriving fully in your heart space, expansive and big. Now exhale and send your breath upward, passing through your upper chest area, your neck, your face, and all the way through the crown of your head into the sky as far as you can imagine it.

Keep the feeling of expansiveness, and on your next inhale draw your breath and your energy down from the sky to enter the crown of the head, as if filling your skull, then drawing down into your heart space. Now, breathe normally and feel yourself connected to the deepest part of the earth and the highest place in the sky that you can imagine and see yourself in the middle, vibrating with the energies of earth and sky meeting at your heart.

STANDING SIDE STRETCH

Stand with your feet hip distance apart and breathe deeply. As you inhale, stretch your arms straight overhead. As you exhale, bring them down by your side again. Inhale, reach up; and exhale, lowering your arms.

Then inhale your arms up and clasp your hands together with your fingers interlaced and index fingers extended. Relax your shoulders and then go down your back, releasing the tension as you keep breathing full and even. Breathe in and out two more times.

On your third exhalation, bend your upper body to the right. Take five slow breaths. Keep the left side steady, feeling that it's anchored down. Slowly return to the center. Repeat on the left side.

Return to center and exhale, lowering your hands down by your sides. Feel the connection between your lungs and your arms, your breath supporting your movement in every way.

Open your heart wide. You are here.

CONNECT WITH NATURE

Another practice for grounding is to walk around outside
or hike with the intention of touching and connecting with
things on your way. If you are in nature, find a tree to hug and
send your roots down to intermingle with its roots. If you are
on a beach, lie down on the sand. Feel yourself being cradled
by the earth. Send your breath to the length of your back and
connect with your support. If you are indoors—in a home for
example—touch the table, furniture, and walls, feeling the
texture and the softness or hardness of things.

Connect with all that you can see. It all came from the
earth. Take a moment to see and acknowledge this; our
acknowledgment shifts our relationship to the things around
us. It roots us in a sense of gratitude.

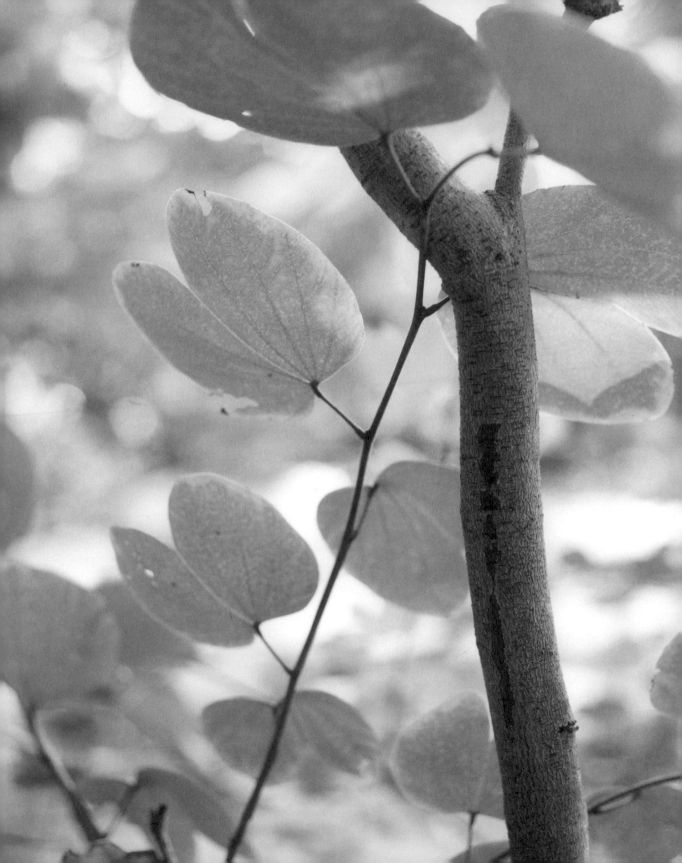

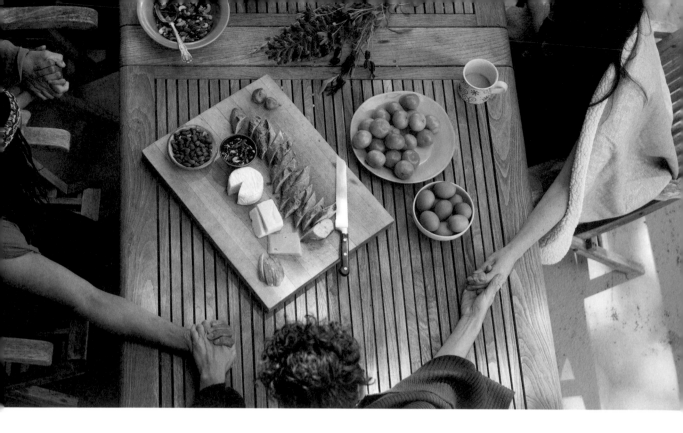

Eating Meditation

Food can be both celebration and nourishment. For many
people food is associated with hunger, guilt, or worry. You
can choose to eat with awareness for your whole retreat, and
it will transform every aspect of your retreat and change the
way you eat when you return. We offer some simple healthy
recipes in the back of the book that can be made with
little effort, feed one person or a large group, and be eaten
throughout the day.

Start your meal with thanks

Whether you are alone or with others, start your meal by giving thanks. Say thank you in whatever version and tradition works for you. In our retreats, we say,

> Thank you for this food,
> which is the gift of the earth
> and much hard work.
> May all people have enough to eat.

Eat in silence for the first ten minutes of your meal

When you eat in silence, you focus on the pleasure of eating. This means not talking to others or on the phone, not reading or listening to the radio while you eat. Just notice and enjoy your food.

Consider having your main meal in the middle of the day

Try eating your largest meal of the day at midday. This supports digestion and ease in the body. You may find you rest better if you don't have a big meal before going to bed. A large midday meal also helps your body process the food and nourishment that it receives.

Have a good time preparing your meal, eating your meal, and cleaning up. Do these things slowly, with gratitude and attention. They can be a joy.

Make each meal beautiful

Your meals don't have to be fancy. Sometimes the simplest food is the best. However, eating is a celebration. Add candles, flowers, good company, or, after your first ten minutes of silence, your favorite music.

Mindful eating means simply eating or drinking while being aware of each bite or sip.
—Thich Nhat Hahn

Play

A retreat doesn't have to be solemn. Play games, put on music, write, and read for fun, and make sure you have time for lightness. If you're with a group, try games to break the ice.

One enjoyable game is called Two Truths and One Little Lie. It gives everyone an opportunity to get to know each other a little better, to find out something that they didn't know before. Also, you have an opportunity to tell an outlandish fib. But don't be too outrageous, or you won't fool anyone.

Two Truths and One Lie

Everyone gets a chance to say three things about themselves, with one thing not being true. Your people have to guess which one is the lie. This can be really challenging if your folks know you well. This game may have you remembering forgotten experiences or talents.

The Metaphor Game

This game works best with five or more people. One person, the Guesser, closes their eyes, the others pick a subject by pointing to someone in the room (it could be the Guesser). The Guesser is then told to open their eyes and has to guess who has been chosen by asking each person one metaphor about the chosen person, for example:

o   If this person were a piece of fruit, what kind of fruit would they be?

o   If this person were the weather, what weather would they be?

o   If this person were an article of clothing, what article of clothing would they be?

After going around the circle and asking the questions, the Guesser has one chance to guess which of the people present is the one being discussed.

Camera

This is mostly a nonverbal game, which can make a nice break and works best with at least four to six people. Have people pair up, with one person in each pair going first as the Camera and the other person as the Leader.

The leader takes the Cameraperson, whose eyes are closed, outside or to a new environment, leading them gently by the hand. When the Leader finds something interesting, beautiful, or unexpected, the Leader positions the Cameraperson in front of that thing and says "Open." The Cameraperson opens their eyes and looks at the thing, just noticing and absorbing it, for five seconds, and then closes their eyes again. The leader then leads the Cameraperson to two more things for them to look at before the two people switch roles.

At the end, the pairs can take fifteen minutes to either write about or draw one of the things they saw.

Rejoicing in ordinary things is not sentimental or trite. In fact, it takes guts.
—Pema Chödrön

Ritual Bath

Consider a ritual bath each day of the retreat. A ritual bath is different from a regular bath. Unlike a regular bath, don't use soap, shampoos, or bath oils. A ritual bath is to support energetic clarity.

Over time, we accumulate energetic dirt and grime as well as physical dirt and grime. It is important to clean our energetic body as well as our physical body. Sometimes the heaviness, unease, or cloudiness that we feel may be from carrying around accumulated energies from people, conversations, our own thoughts, and what is happening around us .

Release, open up and refresh with a ritual bath.

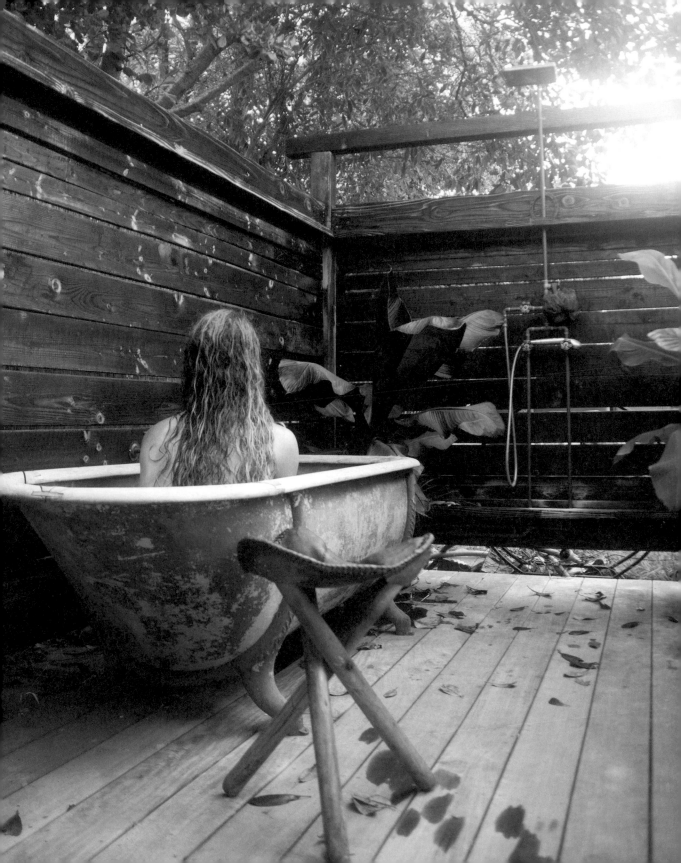

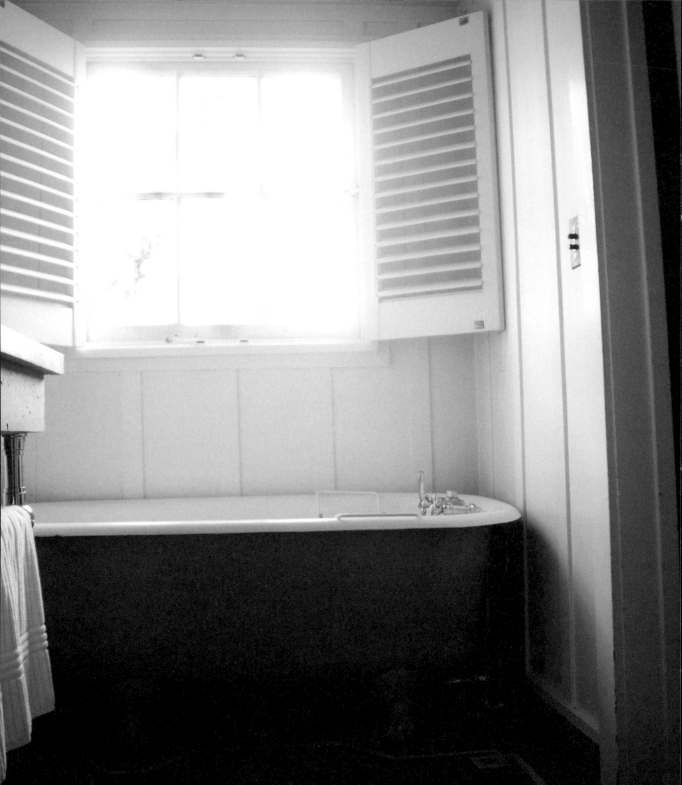

DAY ONE CLEANSING SPIRIT BATH

This is a perfect bath for the first day or night of your long weekend.

Put the ingredients together in a pot and bring to a boil.

Boil for about 3 minutes.
Remove from the heat and steep for 30 minutes.
Remove the sage leaves.
Pour into bath water.

This bath is for clearing the energy of people, places, and things. It is not about "bad or good energy," it is about keeping clear the energetic field that we are.

Give yourself a sesame, almond, or jojoba oil massage after your bath, lovingly rubbing the oil onto your body in circular motions toward the heart, from the bottoms of your feet to the top of your head. Rub a little oil onto your forehead with the tips of your fingers. This quiets the mind.

Afterward, get into your favorite comfy clothes and enjoy a deep sleep.

6 White Sage Leaves in about 8 cups of water

1 cup of Epsom salts

1 tablespoon baking soda

1 teaspoon sea salt

Deep Rest and Relaxation

Rest is a large part of the retreat process. Rest and sleep nourish us.

Deep rest allows us to awaken to ourselves.

We do a lot of things to make ourselves be awake, to be present, to participate in whatever situation we are in. Deep rest is one of our most powerful healers.

Deep rest honors all of the cycles we need for our life and gives us the opportunity to heal whatever imbalance we may create. The body is always moving toward healing.

When we wake up from deep rest, we are more complete. We haven't left parts of us behind. We haven't abandoned the parts of ourselves that want and need rest.

Bring to mind a vision of tomorrow. Imagine yourself waking and the practices that you will engage in. See yourself at ease and fully rested. Decide for your tomorrow, tonight.

If you enjoyed the sitting meditation on arrival, bring it into your evening practice as well. Sit for five minutes before you go to bed for a sumptuous sleep. Lay down anything that has happened in the day. Let the day itself go. Release it and clear space. Allow yourself to be present for this one glorious life by being present one moment at a time.

Let the power of this transition from day into night release your past. When you lay your head on your pillow tonight, choose to feel lighter and clearer.

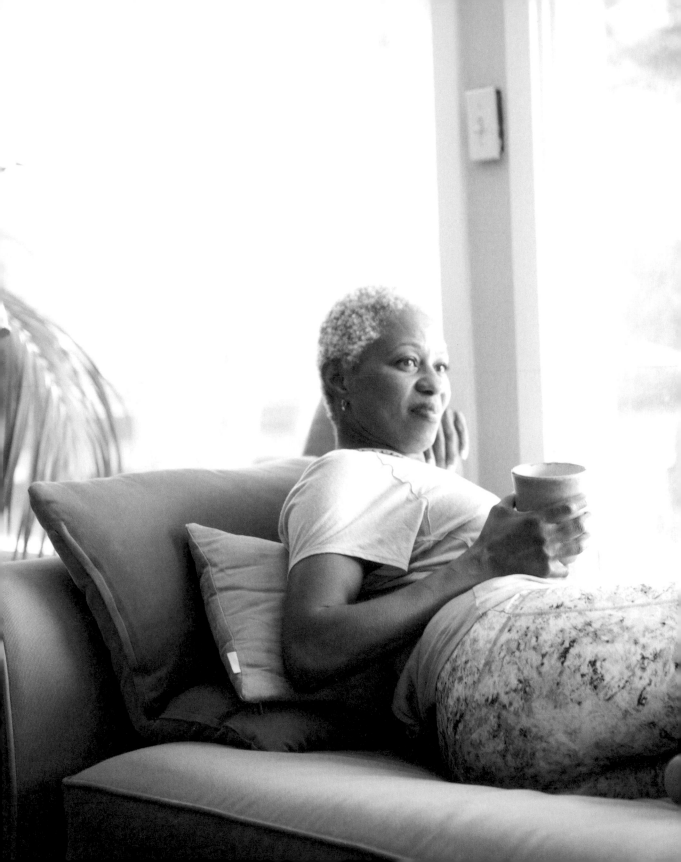

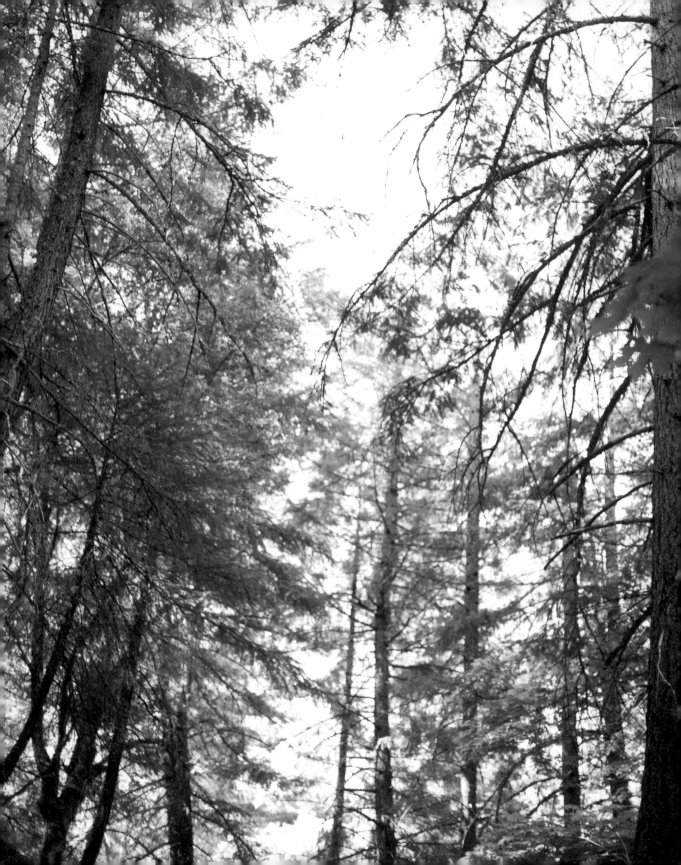

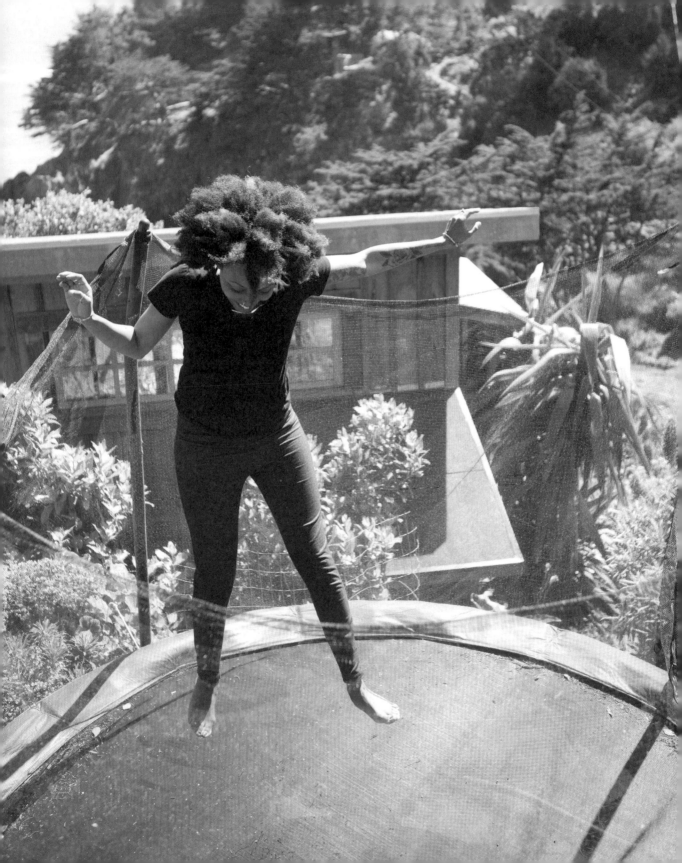

Waking Up to Gratitude

Good Morning Stretch

Writing Your Go-to Story

Hike or Walking Meditation

Self-care and Other-care

Journaling

Storytelling and Sharing

Dance Party

Ritual Bath II

DAY 2

Reclaiming Your Volition

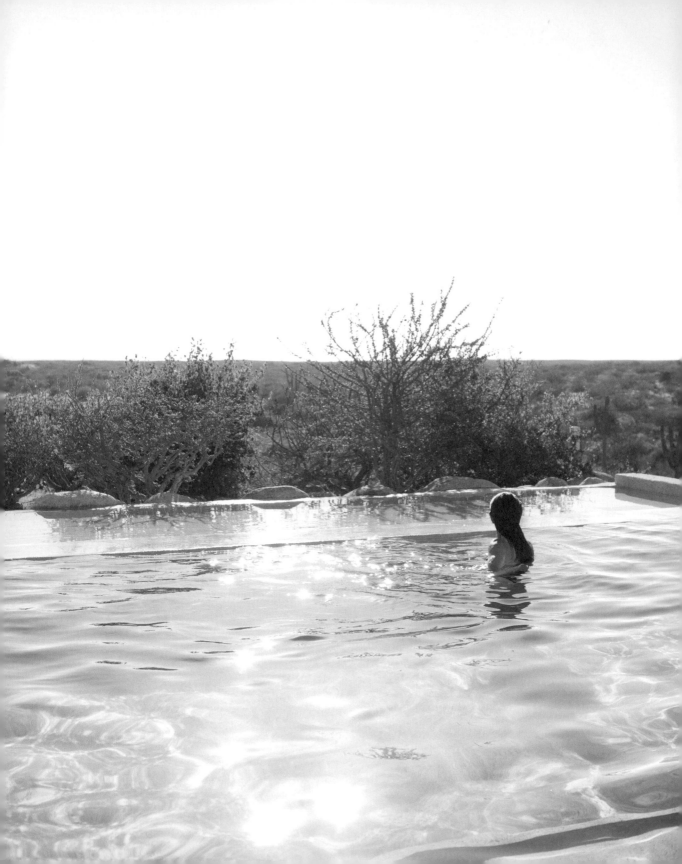

Waking Up to Gratitude

Who will you *be* on this day? The difference between being and doing is that you can't check off being. It is a state of mind and heart. Upon waking up you may go into automatic mode as you get up and start doing—getting right up out of bed as if you have somewhere to go; checking your phone, your clock, your partner, the coffee pot, the paper.

Waking up is about listening and hearing if there was something communicated to you in the night in a dream or in a message that came through; and it's about being still long enough for that message to actually come forth.

There is a very thoughtful, easy way of moving from sleep to gratitude. Whatever comes to mind, I am grateful for, mindfully moving into the day wrapped in a blanket of gratitude. As your feet hit the floor, notice your breath. Does your body feel good and easy or a bit achy? No judgment, just noticing. Gratitude for your body in whatever way it is showing up. As we notice, we begin to have a relationship with our thoughts. Is what we are thinking kind and loving? If it is not, shift to something that is. Shift your thoughts to support your body, your spirit, your being.

Sometimes this is easy. On the first day, it can be a challenge. To be honest, it is always a bit of a challenge. And it is worthy of our effort. It is a lifelong practice. It takes compassion to be with ourselves in a way that is loving and honoring.

Nothing is impossible.
The word itself says "I'm
possible!"
—Audrey Hepburn

Allow the pace of the first day to be slow, slow enough to truly see that everything is a blessing. Every*thing* and every-*one* is a blessing. If you go into the *doing* too quickly, then you'll miss the opportunity.

Today you may feel more rested, or you may feel you need more rest. Sometimes when we finally slow down, our body takes it as a sign to reveal how tired it really is. Listen. If more rest is wanted, give it to yourself guilt-free. This is the point, restoration. Easy walks and good conversations with others or with yourself.

Give yourself the mornings. Align yourself with what you truly desire for your day. Even if it just consists of deep breaths and gratitudes. That's enough.

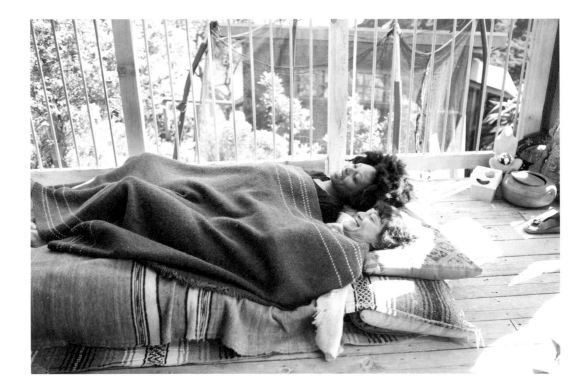

TEN GRATITUDES

Our Gratitudes

Pause before getting up. Let yourself languish in bed. Yawn and stretch and then yawn and stretch again, while bringing your gratitudes to mind. Some of ours are listed at right.

You can also create your own gratitudes. Let them rise up from within.

Allow the Ten Gratitudes to be the foundation for your rising out of bed in the morning. As you get up, slowly feel yourself into your body. Is there something that you are able to hear in this moment as you sit up and listen? Is there a message that is coming forth from a dream or from within your body that hasn't been able to be heard or felt until now?

Sometimes our bodies literally wait until there seems to be space enough in our awareness, until there is a break in our pattern of doing, to speak to us. Our bodies just keep going without what they need because we keep pushing through.

Begin this practice of listening to you, about you.

Let your first drink be warm water with a little lemon. This gently wakes the system rather than jolting it awake like coffee does. You'll want to stay in as much of the half-awake, drowsy place as possible for meditation, when the mind hasn't quite latched on to stories or begun to navigate the day yet.

1. I'm so grateful to open my eyes on a brand new day

2. Grateful for breath in my body

3. Grateful for my bed

4. Grateful for the health of my body

5. Grateful for the day however it's showing up: rainy, sunny, clouds, wind, snow

6. Grateful for all of the abundance, delight, and surprise I know I will experience this day

7. Grateful for a beautiful sleep

8. Grateful for my pillow that supports my head and neck

9. Grateful for my house and the land that it's on

10. Grateful for all of my friends and family (name specific people who come to mind)

Good Morning Stretch

Just because you're awake doesn't mean you have to get up. Take time to recall any dream you had or any question you may have posed right before sleep in the hope that your subconscious mind could take it in while you slept. Take a moment to listen. Remember the gift of quiet and stillness, and as you get up stay in that quiet place.

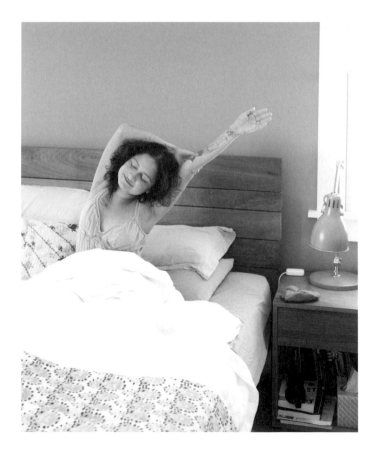

HEART OPENER STRETCH

Stand with your feet about hip width apart, knees soft,
not bent but soft. Clasp your hands behind your back and
breathe deeply into your heart, expanding more and more
with each inhalation. Draw your chin in slightly toward your
chest. Draw your belly in slightly and root the tailbone down
toward your feet. Soften your shoulders and then slide your
shoulder blades down your back.

On an exhale, fold forward. Keeping your hands clasped,
breathe easy and slow for three full breaths.

Release your hands and arms toward the floor and hang for a
moment.

Then bring your hands to your hips, slide your shoulder
blades down the back and towards each other, and inhale as
you come up to standing.

Rotate the hips around, to the left a few turns, then to the
right a few turns.

Shake your body out.

As you move from breakfast into the day, feel your way. You may have made plans for a hike, a walk, for cracking open that book you've so wanted to read, or you may feel that you could go back to bed and close your eyes for another hour or so. Remember, this is your day. Listen to yourself outside of the day-to-day. It may look different from what you had thought or planned. Let that be okay. Be compassionate with those voices or parts of you that say you need to be doing something or sticking to "the plan." Gently redirect your thoughts, reminding yourself to *be*.

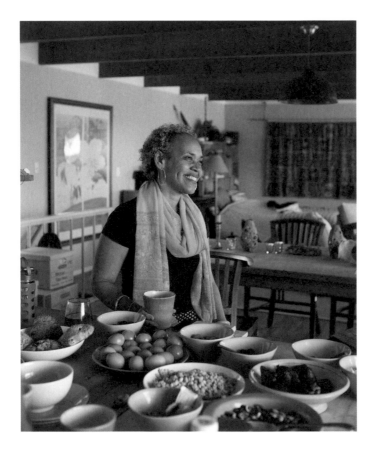

Writing Your Go-to Story

After breakfast and stretching, consider going deeper into a creative project. One option is to write your go-to story. There are stories that we have running in our minds about ourselves. What do you say to yourself about you? Is it loving and supportive? Would you say these things out loud or to a beloved child or friend? If the answer is no, consciously change the thought, the tone, the words to something that you would say to someone you deeply love. It is a practice. This is a beautiful way to begin to shift the thoughts you have about yourself.

There is no greater agony than bearing an untold story inside you.
—Maya Angelou

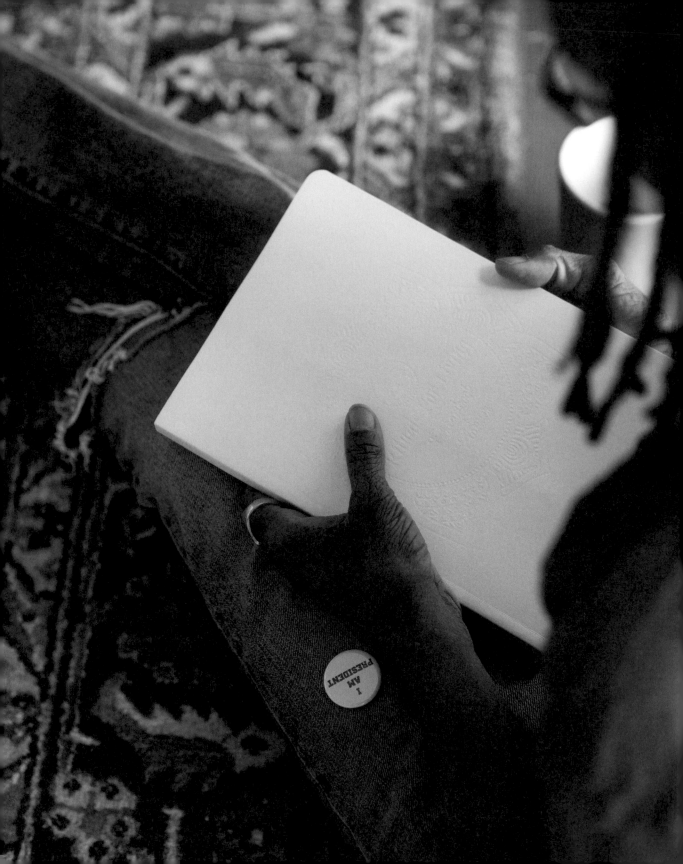

Write your go-to story today as if you were writing to someone you loved deeply. Write a love letter to your body. Have you fallen out of love with any part of yourself? Fall back in love today. Reclaim all parts of you. You are a gorgeous, divine being.

It may be helpful to see yourself as a young person. Imagine the child or the teenager in you or imagine someone you love. Imagine you are using that tone, and write your story.

Tell yourself the truth about your loveliness. Take up a pen or pencil and your journal and write a new story about yourself. This may be easy or you may find places of resistance or not believing. Write it anyway. Work the muscle of loving yourself on paper. Fake it till you make it. We don't always arrive at our healing in one leap. We might need some convincing, and even then most of us just have to jump in.

You can write this as if you were writing a letter to yourself. If you don't know where to begin, start with this line: "Dearest, I've been meaning to tell you . . . ."

Or you can write about yourself in the third person, as if telling a story. You can start with this line: "Once upon a time, there was a . . . ." Make yourself the protagonist of your story. Enjoy the storytelling process.

Hike or Walking Meditation

Spend some time outside in your environment. Whether you are going for a hike or a walk, walking meditation outdoors is a way of being present for every beautiful step on this abundant earth. Notice every part of your body that you employ to move one step forward and then the next, following your breath, focusing entirely on what you are doing and being.

Simple is best. Walk in beauty, look up at the sky, and let be all that there is. Let your thoughts float by like clouds with a gentle wind moving them along.

Your morning practice sets the tone for the day. Presence is the state in which everything comes into focus. You can see more clearly, hear your inhale and exhale, and feel the rhythm of your heartbeat. Feel your arms swing as you walk and notice where your eyes fall and what you see. Then focus more, not a hard focus but a tuning in. What are you really seeing? Meditation is presence. You can be present anywhere and for anything. As you walk, notice which parts of your body move first. What part of the foot connects with the earth first? As you breathe, what are your senses picking up—the smell of the environment, the woods or the water? Is it dry or moist? Is there a breeze, or is there a quiet, a stillness? Walk, breathe, notice, take a picture with your eyes. Feel ease in your body as you move, focus on the spaciousness and expansion from within with each breath. Each breath is a healing. Move in time and in tune with yourself. Presence is in awareness of your breath.

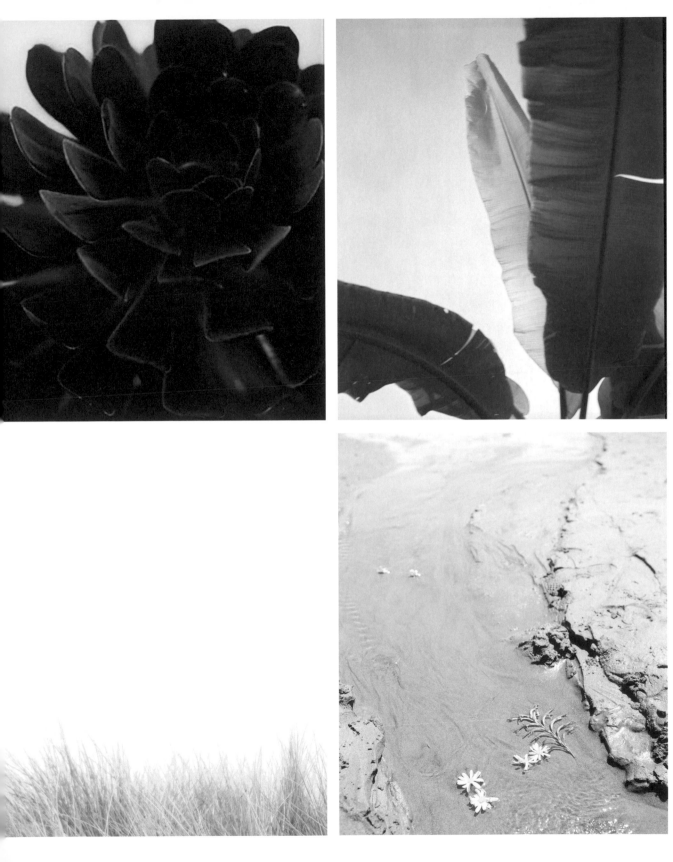

WALKING MEDITATION by THICH NHAT HANH

Walking mindfully on the earth can restore our peace and harmony, and it can restore the earth's peace and harmony as well. We are children of the earth. We rely on her for our happiness, and she relies on us also.

If you look deeply, you can see all the worries and anxiety people imprint on the earth as they walk. Now we have to learn to walk again. Notice each breath and the number of steps you take as you breathe in and as you breathe out. Pay close attention to each breath and each step. Walk slowly, with joy and ease. Let go of your worries and anxieties.

The seed of mindfulness is in each of us, but we usually forget to water it. To have peace, you can begin by walking peacefully. Everything depends on your steps.

*You are the sky. Everything
else is just the weather.*
—Pema Chödrön

Self-care and Other-care

Truly taking care of ourselves is different from paying someone else to take care of us or indulging in something that might leave us feeling worse later. Truly taking care of ourselves involves slowing down enough to pay attention to whatever we are feeling, to acknowledge our exhaustion, or worry, or joy, or fear, or whatever we are feeling. Taking care of ourselves in this way, we act from the recognition that if we are to continue to give out our energy and insight and care to the world, we need to replenish and nurture ourselves.

Spending an afternoon with a few good friends, we can interact in a way that nurtures, supports, and restores us, and reminds us that we can rely on ourselves and each other.

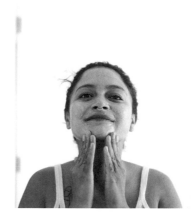

Rachel:

I grew up without electricity or hot water, so the way
we took care of ourselves was often by means of a steam
bath, or a "sweat" as we called it, with cornmeal to soften
the skin.

When we got too hot, we'd run into the creek, or in win-
ter we'd wash our faces with snow. I loved the feeling
of being with other people who I cared about, singing and
sweating. I would always come out of the sweat feeling as if
I was in a completely new moment.

I'm a sucker for any good-smelling lotion, potion, or
scrub. Making scrubs for myself and others is a way to
remind people that they are worthy of care. I've brought
these homemade lotions and balms to protests, retreats, on
work trips, to conferences, and camping. I can be covered in
dirt, sweat, and exhaustion, but if I'm smelling and feeling
good, anything feels doable.

HOMEMADE FACE SCRUBS AND FOOT BATHS

A simple natural face mask and body scrub can be a way to treat yourself without spending money. You are taking care of yourself in a way that feels and smells good. If you're taking a retreat with friends, this is also a way to practice taking care of each other and deepening your relationships.

Oatmeal and Honey Face Mask

Oatmeal is gentle, exfoliating, and moisturizing. It's also naturally anti-inflammatory, so it's perfect for sensitive or itchy skin. Honey is also moisturizing and soothing.

You don't need to cook the oatmeal, but you do need it to be finely ground. If you buy the oats for cooking, you'll need to put them through a blender or Cuisinart to get the more flour-like texture you'll want for the mask. For either mask, let it stay on your skin for 10–20 minutes before rinsing.

MOISTURIZING MASK

1 cup oats

½ cup honey

then add ¼ cup yogurt

FOR OILY SKIN

1 cup oats

¼ cup honey

¼ cup lemon juice.

For either mask, adjust the consistency until you have a paste that you can smooth on.

Sugar or Sea Salt Scrub

No cooking is required. Sugar and salt both work to rejuvenate the skin, though sugar is a little gentler, so use sugar if you are using for your face or other sensitive areas, and use salt only for feet and heels.

1 cup pure cane sugar or
1 cup sea salt

½ cup olive or almond oil

1 teaspoon lavender oil

    Mix ingredients together.

    Adjust the consistency until you have a paste.

    Use on feet, elbows, or anywhere there is rough skin.

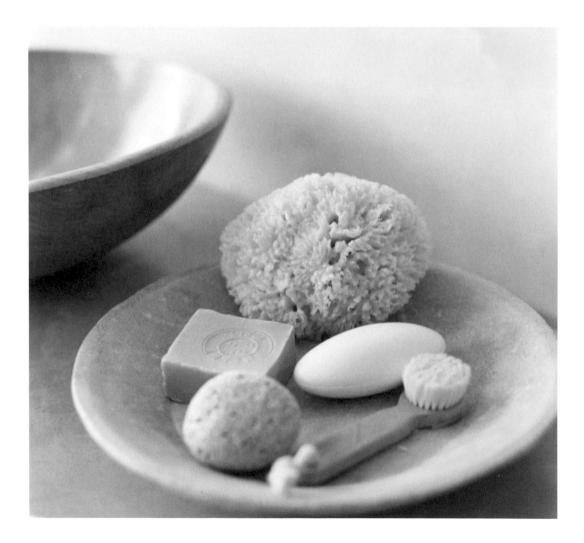

DEEP LISTENING

One way to take care of ourselves and each other that requires no equipment or recipe is Deep Listening. This is a practice of listening to another (or to ourselves) for a set amount of time without judgment or giving advice. If you are in a group, pair up in twos or in groups of three. Agree on a set time (10 minutes works well) and that everything said will be confidential for that session and not discussed afterward without the specific agreement of the person talking. The key piece of this is that, as the active listener, you are fully engaged in listening without commenting or inserting yourself into the experience. Even if you want to insert yourself in a positive way, by encouraging or empathizing, that takes away from deeply listening with enough space for the person to feel truly heard. Try it.

Decide who will listen first.

Set the timer.

One person talks and the other person just listens, for the sole purpose of listening.

The person who is listening doesn't look at her watch or make suggestions or give feedback. She just listens.

Love is our hope and our salvation.
—bell hooks

When the timer goes off, take a one-minute break, either stretching or looking around, and then set the timer for the second person's turn. Again, while you are the listener, you just listen, without judgment.

If you are alone, practice deep listening with yourself. Have a notebook and pen nearby. Set the timer, close your eyes and see what you hear as you listen to yourself. When you hear something, write it down in your notebook without doing anything about it or judging it, and then continue to listen. When the timer goes off, read over what you have written.

Not everything that is faced can be changed, but nothing can be changed until it is faced.
—James Baldwin

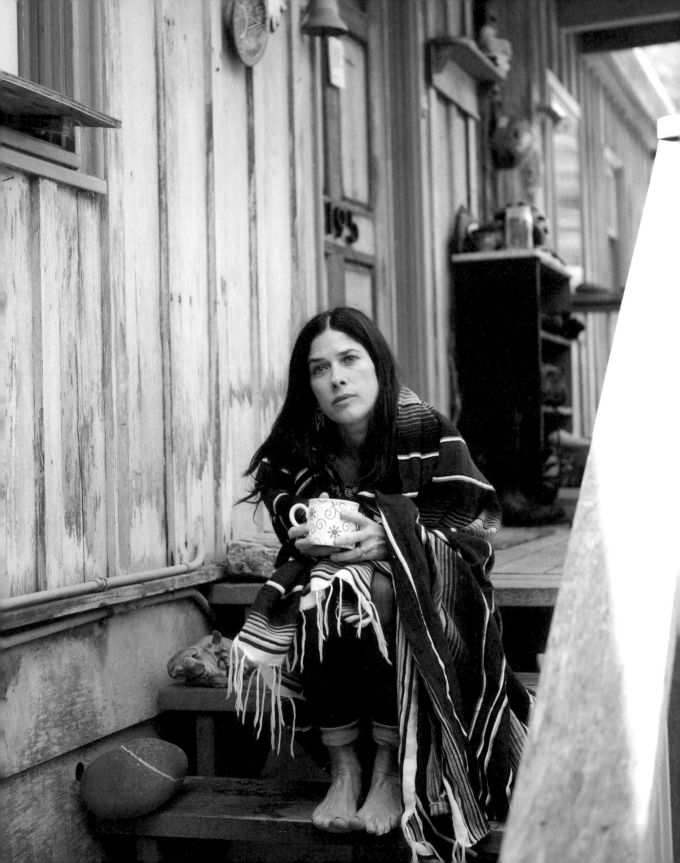

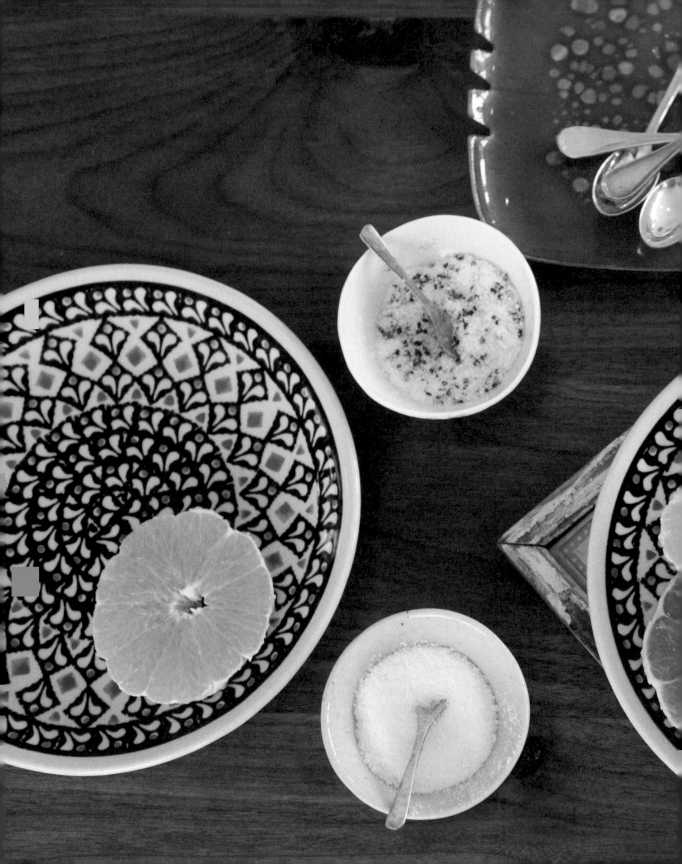

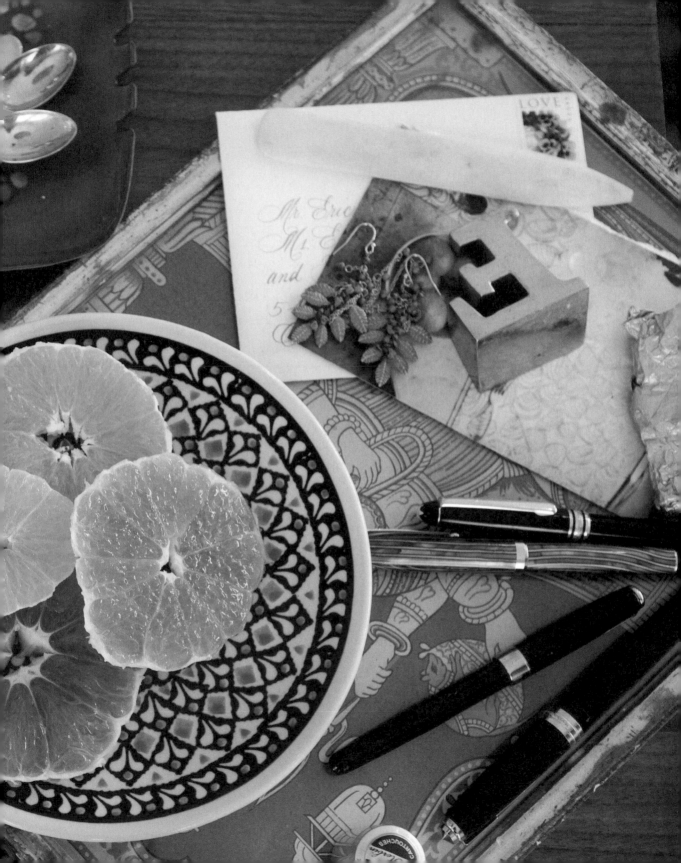

Journaling

Journaling is a powerful way to get whatever you are experiencing, thinking about, and feeling out and on paper. Once we write something and bring it outside of ourselves, we begin to have a different relationship to it. It is a way to track how you are and who you have been over a period of time. Journaling is a way to release the day or an experience so that you may look back on it with some clarity. You can also leave things there in the journal that you no longer need to chew on or carry. When things are moving around in our heads and hearts, we can choose to leave them right there on the page. You can write your journey with something and how you got through it, so you can see from where you've come and how you've arrived to the place where you are. You can log things that you loved and things that you would do differently. It's a check-in of sorts, too. A pause.

If you are not sure where to start, it can be helpful to use prompts or questions that you can answer. You might choose to write at a particular time of day or whenever the feeling arises. Journaling can help in looking back to see your movement and growth in particular areas or to see the places where you may want to have more. When you write, just write—no editing while you are getting your thoughts out. Let them flow freely and see what comes through. When you write without the editor, other possibilities become available. You can still get the facts down and keep it soft around the edges for flow.

Keep it simple; there is no right or wrong way to do it. Avoid making this just another thing on your to-do list rather,

Supplies: pen or pencil and a journal. Simple!

Get comfortable. Get alone. If you are inside in a room to yourself, consider locking the door. If you are outside, go far enough away from others that you won't be disturbed.

Here are some simple basic prompts to start you off:

How am I feeling?

What has happened to me today?

What is something I want to remember?

What colors did I see today?

What is something I heard today?

What was I thinking about when I woke up?

What do I see?

Once you begin, don't edit, cross off, or rewrite. The purpose of journaling here is generative—to get the words out, not to get them perfect.

make it a time for respite and introspection. Journaling can be informative in very interesting ways, especially when you do it regularly. You may begin to notice patterns. You may read your journal and surprise yourself at your own insights. Endeavor to keep it private so you can feel free to write whatever comes. Also, let go of thinking that your spelling must be perfect or all the commas need to be in the right place. If you can read it, that's all that counts. Write by hand, it will give you a whole different experience and relationship to your words and how they flow out. Slow is okay; enjoy the process. Again, it is not a *to-do* but a *to be*.

Be in the process of getting to know your amazing self better.

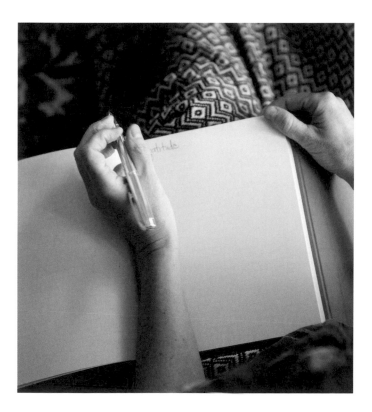

Storytelling and Sharing

Storytelling is a wonderful and fun way to connect with your friends and beloved ones. You can share a story of your own or one from a book that you love, reading aloud with all the drama you want; act it out! Storytelling and sharing are ways to share our past, regardless of whether the story we are sharing is from last week, last year, from our parents or ancestors, or is one we have made up. It is the way that human beings have passed on our history from generation to generation, through oral cultures and traditions. Of course with each ear that heard it, with each imagination it captured, with each person who saw it acted out or retold, it would shift and change a bit with the flourishes and embellishments of the one telling the story. You can tell stories about family or experiences that you've had. We are all such interesting beings.

You can also tell a story that is completely fictional, made up on the spot, taking in clues from wherever you are or whoever is in the room. You can begin a story and then pass it around for each person to add their own piece to the telling. Most of the stories that we see now are on a screen. What are our own stories? What can we pass on through generations that will be told and retold? That has our voice, our facial expressions remembered, that has us in them?

Each day has a story that deserves to be told, because we are made of stories.
—Eduardo Galeano

Richelle:

I still recall the stories that my brother would tell to try
and scare me when we were little and supposed to be asleep.

We had bunk beds and he got the top bunk. So I was clos-
est to the floor and whatever he made up was always lurking
under my bed. I knew that he was just trying to get a rise
out of me, and it worked. I acted like I wanted him to stop,
but I loved every minute of it.

He was my big brother—I knew he'd protect me. I was
grateful when he would laugh at me when he saw my face
stretched and wide-eyed with fear as he looked over the edge
of his bunk. It made me laugh too. Oh, big brothers!

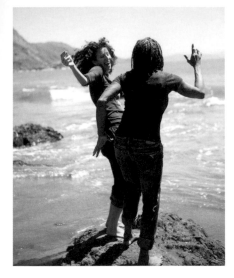
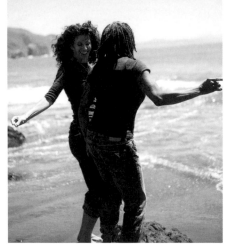
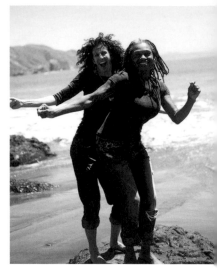
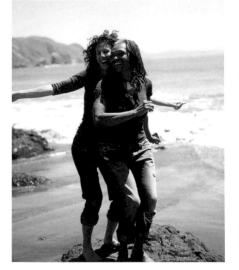
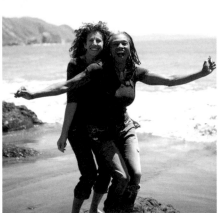
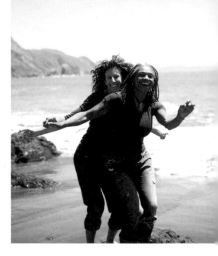
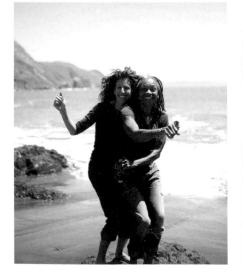
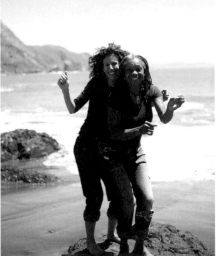
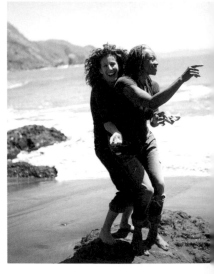

Dance Party

You can have a dance party at your long weekend whether it is a solo retreat, a group of only three or four, or a much larger gathering. Why? Because dancing is an opportunity to reacquaint yourself with joy. It's a great way to get rid of any stuckness in your body and mind. When you're moving, your energy flows. Sometimes we don't know we were stuck until we start to move. Yoga, walking, running, hiking are all great ways to create flow and movement. But there is nothing like dancing to set the body and spirit free. As Martha Graham says, "Dancing is the hidden language of the soul of the body."

Dancing is a balm. Maybe it has healed your body and spirit from real and imagined wounds. Maybe dancing has freed you up emotionally and creatively time and time again. Dancing is a sensory and intuitive activity. We are all sensual beings. What we see, hear, smell, taste, and touch can bring us so much joy. But our receptivity to sensations can get clouded and dulled by life lived while our attention is stuck to a screen and disconnected from our body. We can start to settle for that which is outside of us and think that we can find our true joy in online purchases and quick consumption.

No two people move alike. Explore your own natural movement. When you allow yourself to move, what is within you must come out. You don't have to know what is going to come next as you dance. It just comes. You have your own unique brand of movement, your own rythym, your own beat, your own groove.

To dance is to be out of yourself. Larger, more beautiful, more powerful. This is power, it is glory on earth and it is yours for the taking.
—Agnes De Mille

Connecting to our own body, feeling safe and comfortable in our body, is a kind of freedom. Dancing grounds us in our body and, when we are grounded, we are more powerful in all we do in the world. How we are in our body affects every part of our lives, our families, our communities, our work, and our creativity. Dancing shakes us up, and we all need to be shaken up. Everything withers and dies without love and attention. Dancing is a way to honor and let loose our inherent joy.

Let this be reason enough to put on something you feel good dancing to and begin wiggling. Move those hips, those arms, put on a little Stevie Wonder or Aretha Franklin or David Bowie or whoever makes you feel good and reclaim your life.

Throw off any judgment, any thought that limits you, that has you saying "no" or has you doubting that you can dance. Your movement is your movement and it's perfect! It is love. This can create tremendous healing in places that we may not even know need healing. This energy is boundless. Go ahead and get your dance on!

You are amazing, extraordinary, and powerful.

Be joyful with your body. No judgment; just feel. Remember your magnificence outside of the stories that can keep you held in tightly-packed spaces. Break out! Put on some tunes. Maybe take turns DJing. Put on some of your favorite tunes from back in the day. See if you can remember some of your dance moves. Set yourself free and dance!

I want freedom, the right to self-expression, everybody's right to beautiful, radiant things.
—Emma Goldman

Ritual Bath II

After whatever adventure you chose for the day, take a ritual bath. Let the water carry away anything you are choosing to let go of; let it go down the drain. Wash away judgments, old tired stories, *if onlys* and *what ifs*. Leave the bath or shower feeling lighter.

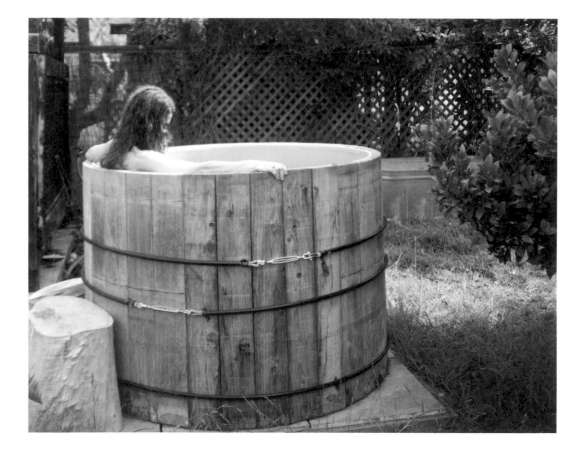

DAY TWO I-LOVE-MYSELF BATH

Draw a warm bath and put in one of the two essential oil combinations below.

Ylang ylang, lavender, and myrrh essential oils
(3–5 drops of each)

or

Clary sage, frankincense, and mandarin
(3–5 drops of each)

Then add:

1 cup Epsom salts

1 handful rose petals

Optional: music

Place the rose petals in the bath just before you get in.
Soak for 20 minutes or until the water cools.

DAY TWO HEALING MYRRH BATH

Draw a warm bath. Add:

> 1 packet unscented oatmeal bath powder, breakng up
> the clumps

> 10 drops myrrh essential oil

Soak until the bath cools.

Pat yourself dry and dress in loose, breathable clothing.

You can substitute the myrrh with 10 drops lavender and 5 drops chamomile.

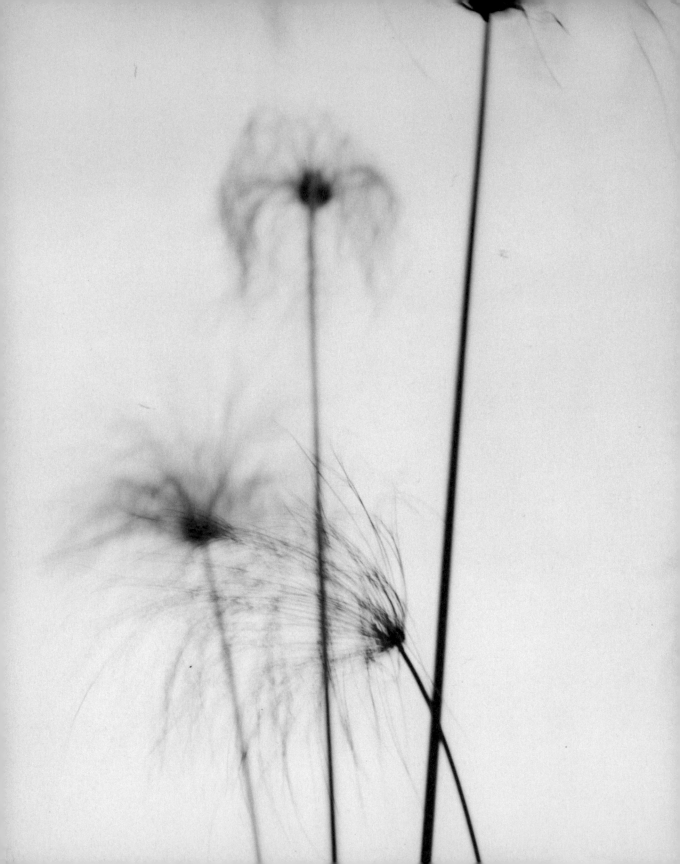

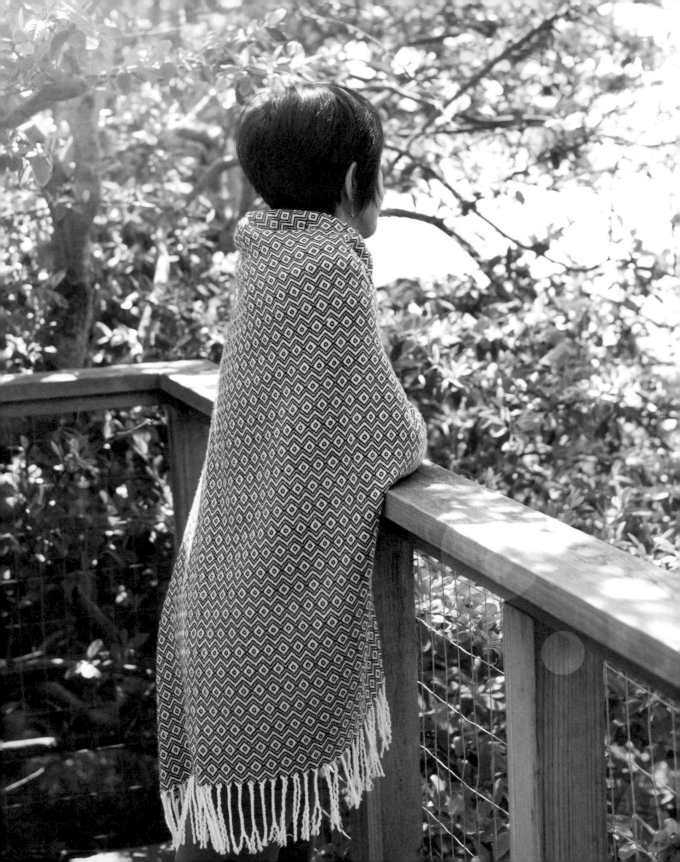

Heart Openers

Vision Board

Hugging/Goodbye Meditation

Turning Toward Home

A Little Long Weekend Every Day

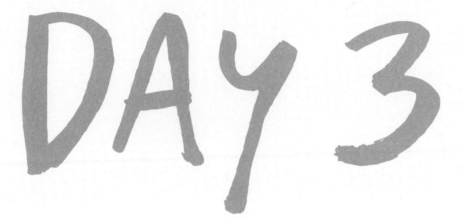

DAY 3

Standing Your Ground,
Opening Your Heart

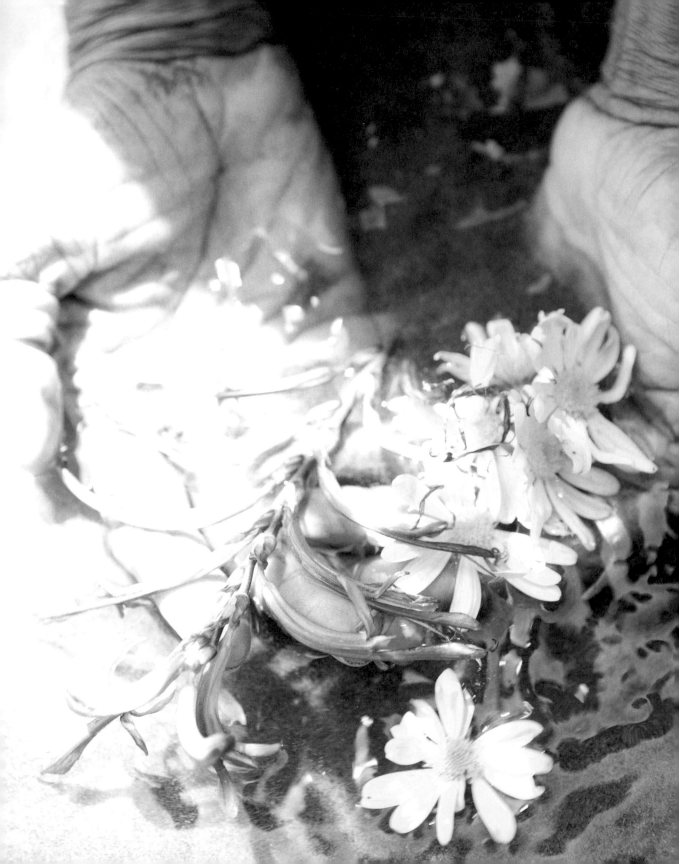

Heart Openers

Day Three calls for you to practice some of the same ways of being, but differently. Different because *you* are different. You now know more about yourself, your desires, how to care for yourself, what is working, and what you can let go of, what you are willing to be so that you can truly restore your body and soul.

After morning practices, after your yummy breakfast, don't rush. Begin the morning with a physical practice before you travel home. Take your time with the Heart Opening practice below, letting your heart revel in the openness and ease.

Often on our last day as the end is coming near, we find ourselves moving away all too soon from the new practices that we have been cultivating over the long weekend. Be aware of this, and instead, go deeper into what you love. Meditate a little longer. Get freer with your dancing, your writing, all of the things you have done and whatever you haven't done that you have saved for today. Turn up the volume, tune in to that voice within. You have more of a relationship to it now. Keep cultivating that. Be with it so much that you recognize it above *all other* voices. Grow and grow that still-small voice of intuition and knowing.

Forget your voice, sing!
Forget your feet, dance!
Forget your life, live!
Forget yourself and be!
—*Kamand Kojouri*

GETTING IN TOUCH WITH YOUR BREATH

Sit on a chair with your feet flat on the floor, knees and feet hip distance apart. Make sure that your knees are in alignment with your hips, not too high or low. Use a pillow or choose a different chair to create this alignment. Bring your hands to your thighs so that your elbows are directly under your shoulders. Draw your belly in slightly with an inhale and lift the heart toward the chin.

Draw your ears back toward the back of your body. This can be a challenging instruction to understand, so here is a way to get there. Jut your chin and head all the way forward, now do the opposite and draw the head and chin all the way straight back, slide forward, now glide straight back, slide forward, glide back and on the last glide back, stay there. The chin is neither tucked nor lifted. Your ears are aligned with your shoulders. This may feel weird because usually our head is forward when we're texting, reading, driving, or on our computer. This position is important to know well and to practice often because it immediately brings ease to the nervous system and the neck.

Begin breathing more deeply into the heart. Fill the lungs and bring awareness to the area of your solar plexus, which is below the heart. Fill the back of the body with breath. Continue to deepen your in-breath and lengthen your out-breath.

Holding your beautiful posture upright, place one hand on your belly, one hand on your heart, and begin deep belly breaths. Relax your abdominal muscles, and slowly inhale through the nose, bringing air into the bottom of your lungs. You will feel your abdomen fill. This expands the lower parts of the lungs. Continue to inhale as your rib cage expands outward, and finally, the collarbones rise. At the peak of the inhalation, pause for a moment, then exhale gently from the top of your lungs to the bottom. At the end of exhalation, contract your abdominal muscles slightly to push residual air out of the bottom of your lungs.

Repeat five times:

My heart is at ease.
I am loved.

Feelings come and go like clouds in a windy sky. Conscious breathing is my anchor.
—Thich Nhat Hanh

GENTLE HEART OPENERS

Stack pillows or folded blankets/towels to make a rectangular stack about 3–5 inches high.

Sit in front of the stack with your bottom on the floor, then lay all the way back with the length of your spine and your head on the stack. Place the soles of your feet together and allow your knees to fall out to the sides. Take a pillow or a stack of blankets or towels and wedge them under your thighs to allow your legs to relax there. Or stretch your legs straight out and put a pillow, blanket, or bolster under your knees. Sometimes you can find just the right size pillow for this on a couch. If this is challenging to do on the floor you can do it on your bed.

Use as many blankets as it takes for complete comfort. Close your eyes, place one hand on your heart, and one hand on your belly.

You can repeat this affirmation just once or repeatedly:

My heart is open and full of grace.
I am safe and at ease.

Relax and breathe for 5 minutes.

Vision Board

One way to preserve and grow the work that takes place this weekend is to create a Vision Board that can act as a visual reminder, when you're back at work or at home, of what you want to remember from your long weekend.

Reflect on how you have grown and create a soul picture of what you have discovered in this time away.

Let this visual represent what you would love to weave into your daily life.

*Nobody sees a flower—
really—it is so small it takes
time—we haven't time—
and to see takes time, like
to have a friend takes time.
—Georgia O'Keefe*

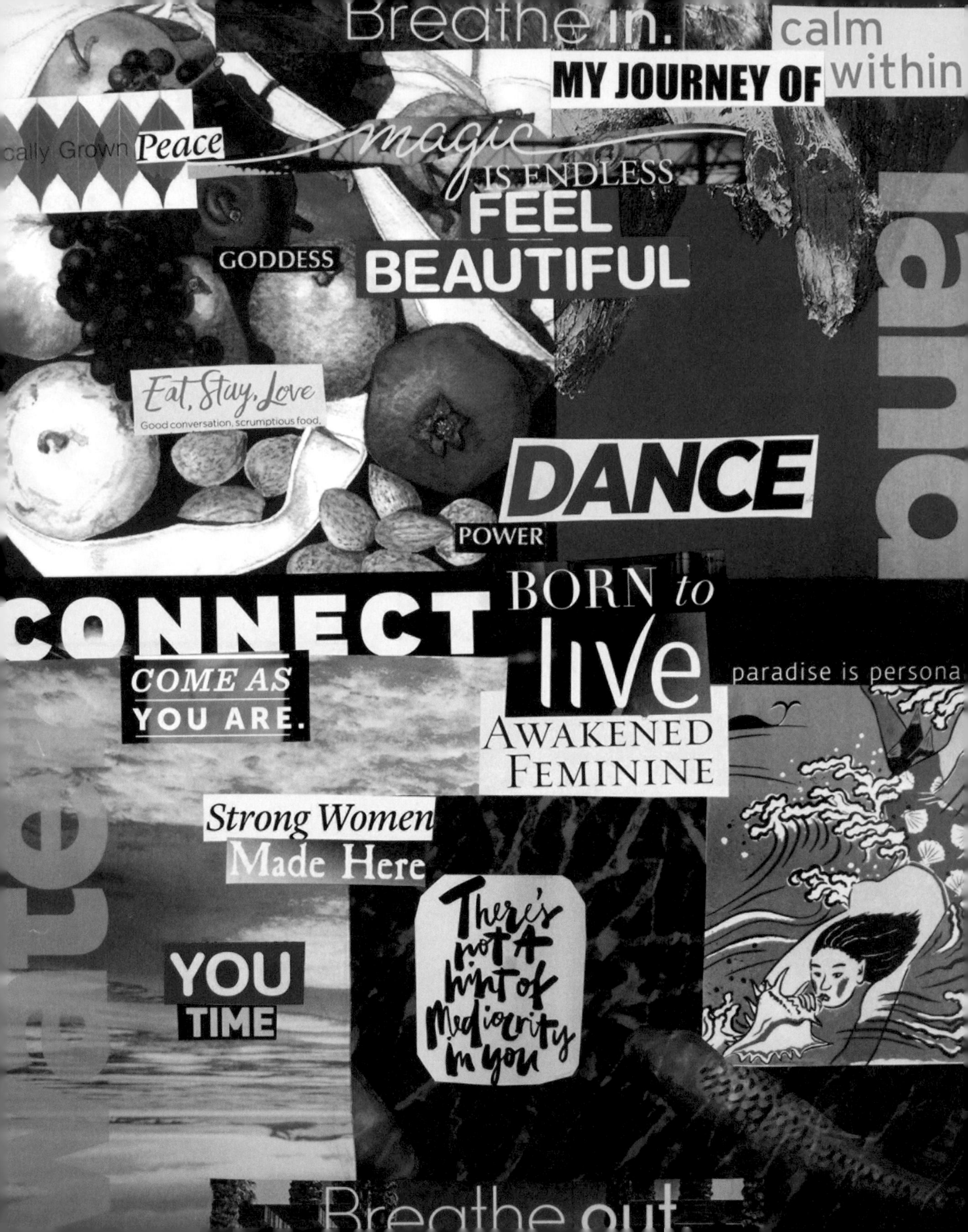

Breathe in.

calm within

MY JOURNEY OF

cally Grown Peace

magic IS ENDLESS

FEEL

BEAUTIFUL

GODDESS

Eat, Stay, Love

Good conversation, scrumptious food.

DANCE

POWER

CONNECT

BORN to

live

paradise is persona

COME AS
YOU ARE.

AWAKENED
FEMININE

Strong Women
Made Here

There's
not A
hint of
Mediocrity
in you

YOU
TIME

Breathe out

VISION BOARD

Get your Vision Board station set up with all of your supplies and then begin looking through the magazines and other materials for images, words, or phrases that inspire you. You'll know when you look at it whether it aligns with a feeling, a knowing, a being, a clarity, an impulse, if it inspires. Maybe it's a picture of a beautiful place, and when you see yourself there, you feel life is fantastic. Choose images that remind you of your highest and best, images and words that remind you of who you are choosing to be, images that remind you of what you are loving about your Long Weekend. Cut them out.

Wait until you have several and can see a direction or theme before you paste them onto your board; this will reveal itself naturally. Once you have a good number of cut-outs, look for background imagery, something to go beneath the images and words—it might be flowers, colors, sky, ocean, or something big and beautiful that reminds you of your Long Weekend or the next one that you will go on—and glue the background on first. Then begin to place your words and images on the board. Don't glue them yet, just place them so you can see where they work best. There will come a moment when you begin to have an idea how your finished vision board will look. It doesn't have to be finished yet; it might be only fifty- to seventy-percent done. Just be sure the main bits are there. Now, take a photo so you know where you've placed everything. Then take everything off the board so only the background is left.

SUPPLIES

_ The board can be whatever size you choose, 8" x 10" or larger. The board can be made of cardboard or wood.

_ Plenty of magazines, newspapers, flyers, cards, anything that might have an inspiring picture or message.

_ A good pair of scissors, or 2 or 3 pairs if you're doing it with others.

_ Glue sticks or hot glue gun.

Begin to glue the pictures onto the board. The picture can help with overlapping images so you know which one to glue down first. Once you begin to glue, it gets even more exciting. More images may come along that you'll want to add, whether in that moment or over time. You can continue to add to your vision board.

This is a living, breathing expression of what you love. This is your Vision. Put it someplace where you can see it every day and step into that feeling it brings you as often as possible. Remember who you are choosing to be. You are this Vision.

This is a place that you can visit daily. Put your vision board somewhere close at hand so you can look at it.

The most important thing about having a vision is that you begin. Now is the moment. Your vision is not for the future but for now. Hold it with an open hand. Begin the process by taking a step. It's like when you had a vision for a long weekend, the first thing you did was to put it on your calendar. What would you love to create in your life that either doesn't exist yet or that you would love to have more of? Love, peace, dancing, work, money, time, a partner? Write it out, create a vision board that reflects the qualities of the life you would love to live. Then live from that state of mind and being every day.

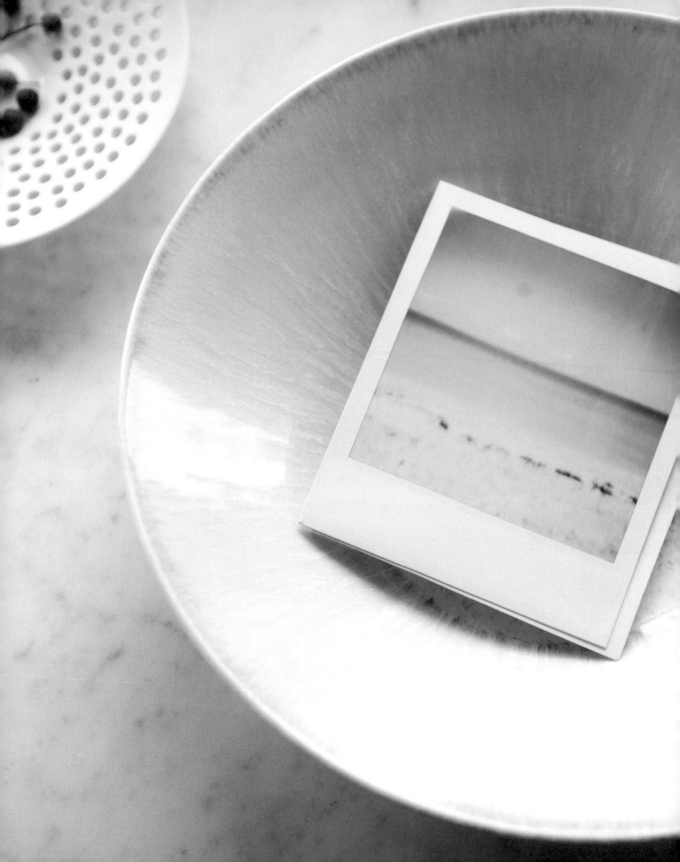

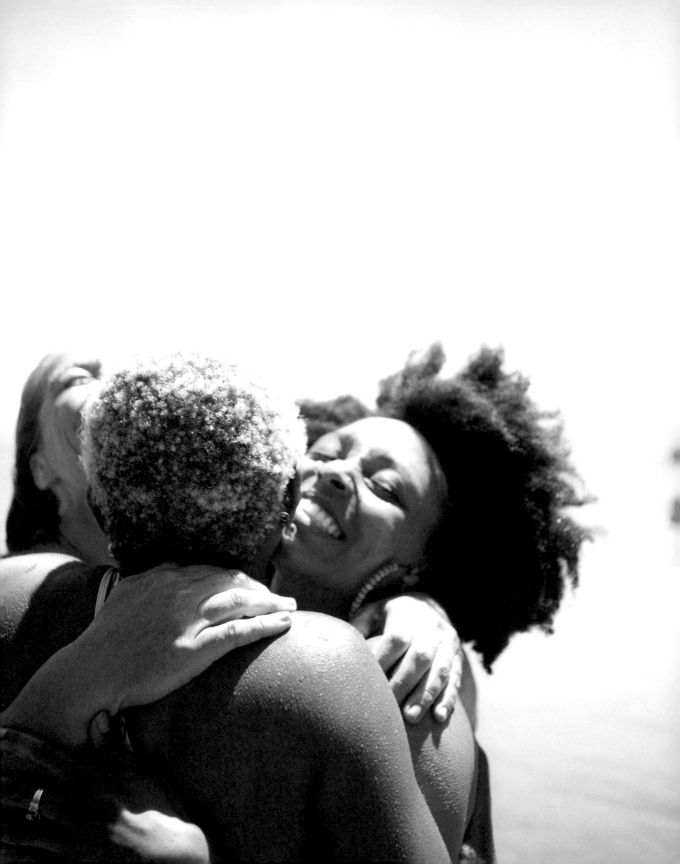

Hugging/Goodbye Meditation

Leaving your retreat can be difficult. Take the time to say goodbye to the time you have had with yourself, and with your loved ones if they are there with you.

Honor the transition by saving time for goodbyes.

I've been absolutely terrified every moment of my life—and I've never let it keep me from doing a single thing I wanted to do.
—Georgia O'Keefe

BREATHING MEDITATION:
HELLO AND GOODBYE

Set up as you would for sitting meditation, but keep your eyes open (just gaze slightly downward). Don't force your breathing or try to modify it in any way as you inhale and exhale.

When you inhale, be aware of the inhalation. Welcome the breath by saying silently in your mind, "Hello." When exhaling, bid farewell to the breath by saying silently to yourself, "Goodbye."

With every inhalation and exhalation, repeat, "Hello, goodbye, hello, goodbye." In this way, you are neither accepting nor rejecting what comes and goes. When the breath comes in, you welcome it with awareness: when the breath goes out, you bid farewell by mindfully letting it go.

You might be wondering what the purpose is of saying "hello and goodbye."

This practice allows us to remember that we are constantly coming and going, forming, dissolving, and changing. As meditation teacher Spring Washam says, "Hello/Goodbye… is the deep understanding that we're here and then we disappear. Things come together for a period and then quite organically dissolve again."

Turning Toward Home

Give yourself a big high five for the wondrous way that you have cared for yourself over the last few days and for your commitment to carry this way of being with yourself forward.

As you leave the space of the long weekend, whether it is your own home or somewhere else, leave with the rituals that you came in with, created, and cultivated.

Feel your feet on the floor. Take three deep breaths. Breathe in long (through your nostrils) and breathe out slowly (through your mouth). Look around you, blessing everything with your gaze. Bring again, to mind and heart, your original intention for your long weekend. Remember who you are *being* and carry this intention and awareness back into your daily life.

It is easy to return return to life as it was before the long weekend. We tend to separate our everyday selves and the life-changing experiences we have during a break or a vacation. Your experience of the long weekend can be different. Ask yourself the question: how can I stay connected to this practice that feeds me? How can I carry this forward with me?

Wait as long as you can to turn toward your life at home, even if you are aready at home. Wait to turn on the phone. Wait to look at your emails. Wait to do these things until you absolutely must do so. And when you do, you will be wholly different and much more present.

This being human is a guest house. Every morning a new arrival.
—*Rumi*

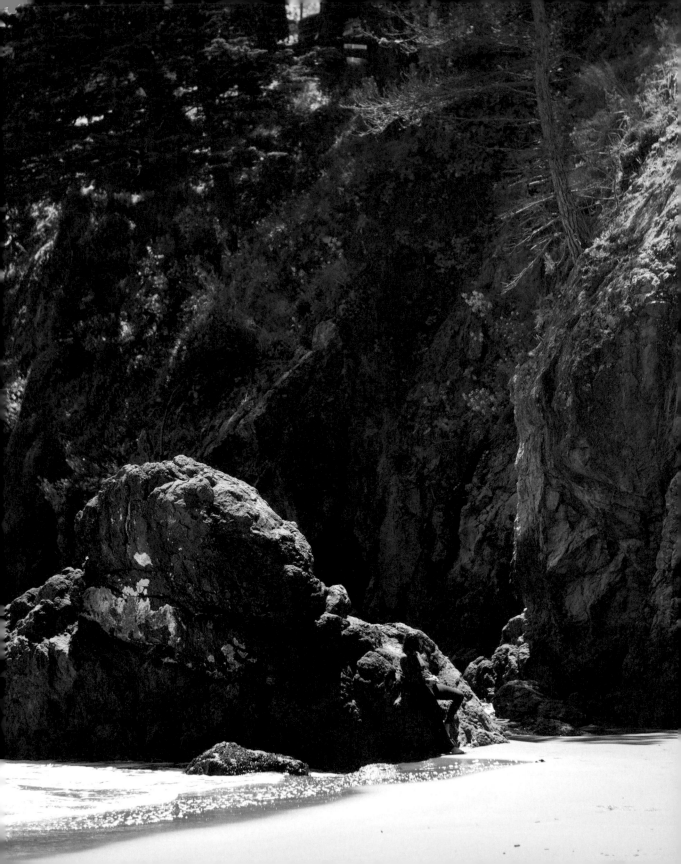

You have plenty of time to get back to your daily life. Stay with yourself. Stay in the energy that you created. Stay in the love that you created for yourself. Stay with the ease and grace of this time of the long weekend. It is profound and powerful to know yourself outside of the day-to-day. To be aware and in alignment with what you would love is to be in-touch with your truest self.

A long weekend is not just about getting away, *it is about transformation*. Every day. What you have created here with yourself is yours. Preserve it; grow it.

Your heartbeat is a kiss that reminds you more than a hundred thousand times a day that you are truly deeply loved.
—Richelle Donigan

A Little Long Weekend Every Day

Take your long weekend back into your daily life.

A wonderful way to start every day is to say gratitudes before your feet hit the floor and you get out of bed.

Take time for that long stretch and a good yawn right there in bed. This is an easy way to wake up the spine, joints, and muscles. Mmmm, deliciousness.

Meditate for five minutes each morning. It's your time with yourself, in silence, before any other voice comes in. Just five minutes. You can meditate longer if you have time, but just five minutes is already golden.

If in under fifteen minutes you have said some gratitudes, have had some good body stretches, and some silence, it's already a *good* day.

What's on your wall, your mirror, your computer screen? Make sure it affirms the truth about how wonderful you are and supports who you know yourself to be deep down.

If you did the walking meditation practice on your retreat, do it now as you walk from one room to another, whether at home, at work, or out in nature.

Take a bath! A sage tea bath will keep clearing energy, and you can throw in the I Love Myself bath here and there.

Keep that playlist on repeat and just dance, dance, dance, DANCE!

Put another long weekend on the calendar.

If we were not so single-minded about keeping our lives moving, and for once could do nothing, perhaps a huge silence might interrupt this sadness of never understanding ourselves.

—Pablo Neruda

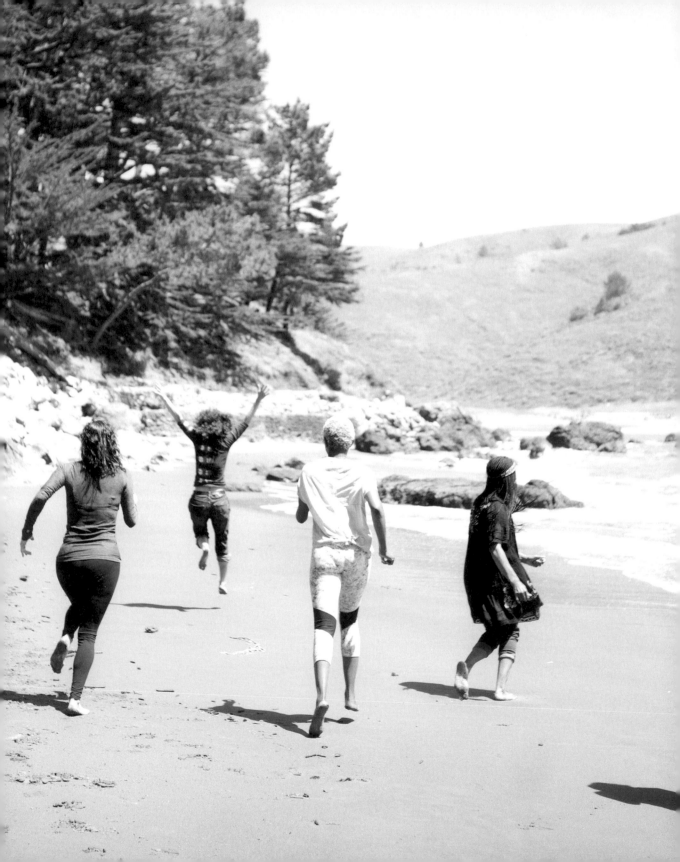

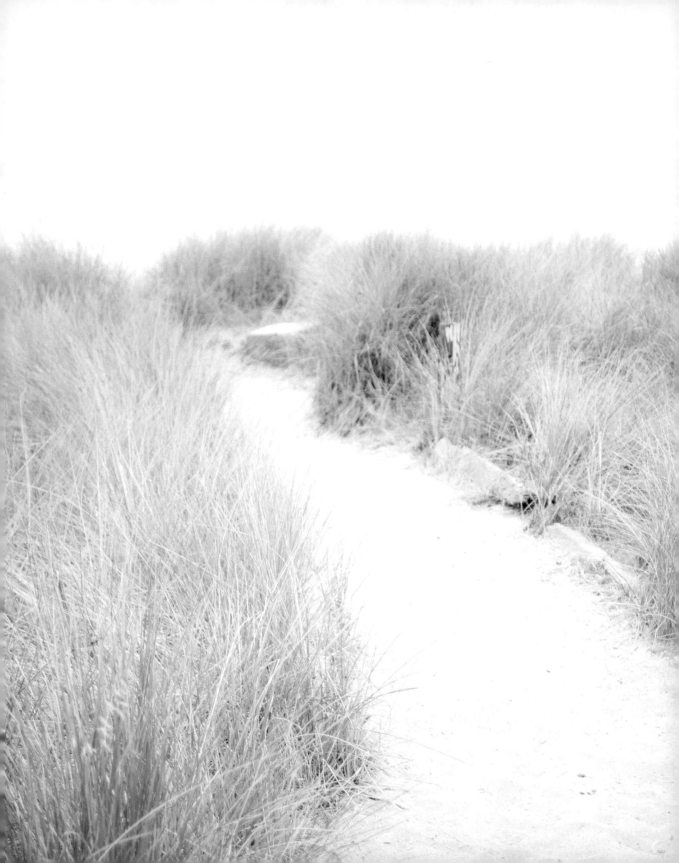

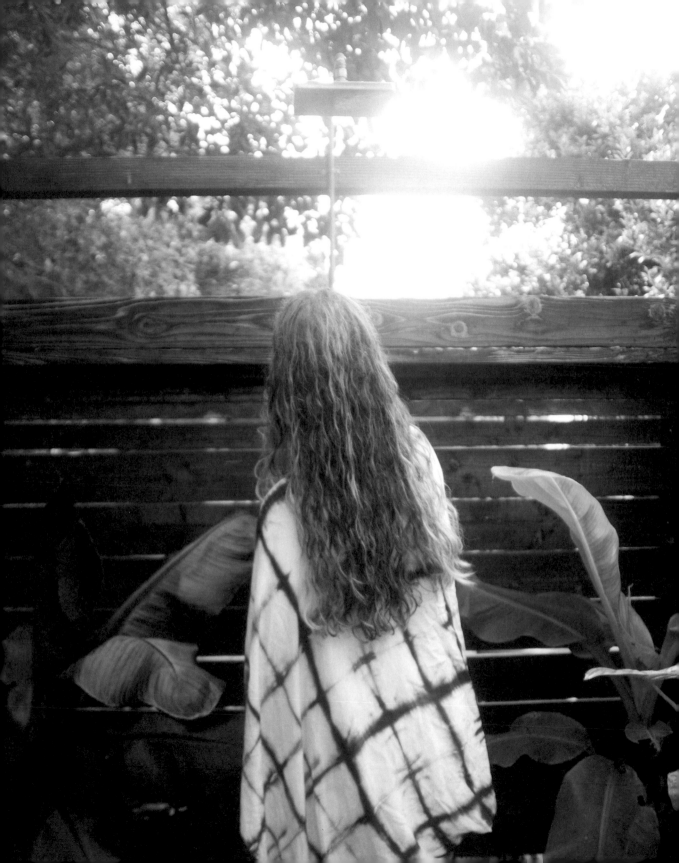

Recipes for Your Long Weekend

Richelle's Affirmations

Playlists

Grocery Lists

Retreat Centers

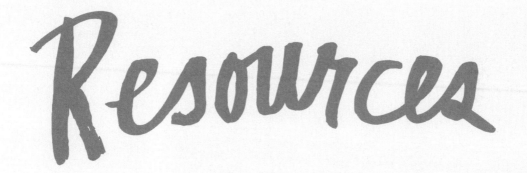

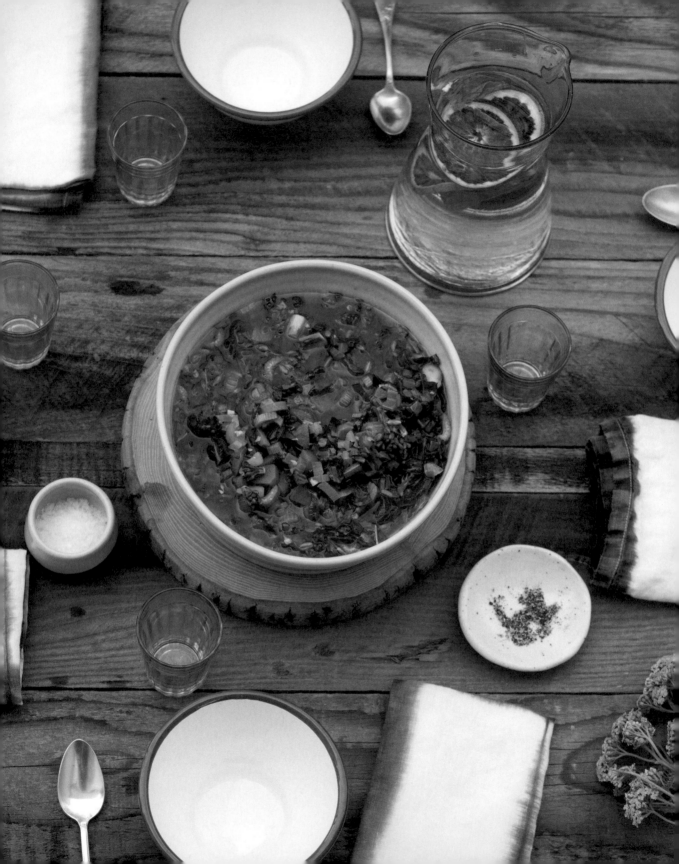

Recipes for Your Long Weekend

Developed by Chef Kelly Foster

These recipes are designed to be plant-based, light, nourishing, conducive to creative activity, and flexible enough to work for a variety of meals (and people). Each recipe here is created for 4–6 people, so expand or reduce the quantities according to your group size.

DRINKS

All-day-long Drinks

- Infused Waters
- Teas

Morning Drinks

- Smoothies

Infused Waters

- strawberries + basil
- strawberries + mint
- cucumber + mint
- cucumber + lemon
- citrus combo of lemon + lime + orange
- grapefruit

Select the fruit you want to use for your infused water. Wash it thoroughly. Whenever possible, buy organic fruit and vegetables. Conventional strawberries, in particular, are sprayed with a lot of pesticides. Next, cut or slice your favorite fruits and place them in a pitcher or glass jar. Then pour some filtered or distilled water over the fruit and place in the refrigerator overnight. The next morning you will awaken to refreshing and flavorful water. Use the above fruit combinations to help you get started. Experiment with various fruits to create different flavor combinations.

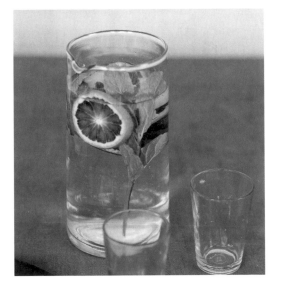

Teas

- mint
- chamomile
- dandelion
- green tea

Mint tea can aid digestion, and chamomile tea can also help to warm and soothe our bodies when we need to rest or relax. Dandelion tea is a great aid in removing toxins from the body.

Store-bought herbal teas are fine; however, if you have access to a garden, you can also pick some fresh mint leaves and pour hot water over them and let them steep for a good 10 minutes before drinking.

If you are trying to take a break from your morning coffee during the retreat, green tea is a nice alternative. It does contain caffeine, but it gives you an even stream of energy instead of the quick up-and-down of coffee.

With any tea, follow the directions on the package for the best brewing results. If you can, drink your tea without any refined sugar.

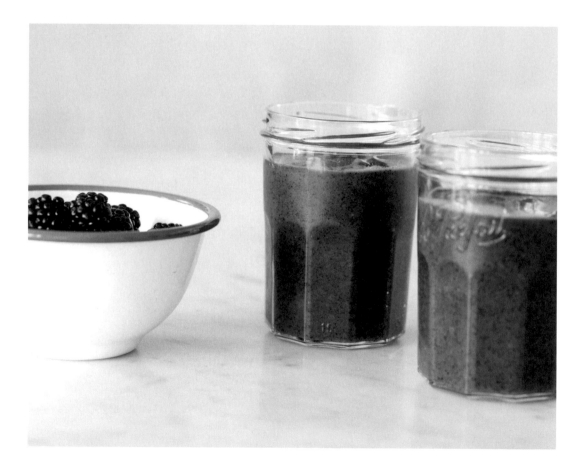

Smoothies are an easy way to begin the day. Frozen or fresh fruit can be used. Frozen fruits are a great because you can find a fairly wide variety in the freezer section of the market and they help make the smoothie cold and add that thick consistency to them.

Smoothies

Antioxidant Smoothie

¾ cup blueberries (fresh or frozen)

¼ cup each strawberries and raspberries, blackberries (or any combination of these, fresh or frozen)

½ to 1 banana. Look for speckles, to ensure ripeness

2 leaves kale (curly or dino kale), cut or chopped after removing stems

2 or 3 pitted dates

1 cup nondairy milk such as almond or soy, or filtered water

Place all ingredients in the blender. Blend on high until all the ingredients are combined. If you do not have a high-powered blender, you may need to switch off your blender a few times to stir the ingredients and help them blend. Once everything is well blended, pour into a glass and enjoy.

Key Lime Smoothie

juice of 1 lime

juice of ½ lemon

½ banana

1 cup nondairy milk, such as almond, hemp, or soy milk

2 or 3 pitted dates

1 teaspoon vanilla flavoring (optional)

Place all ingredients in the blender. Blend on high until smooth. Pour into a glass and enjoy.

Sweetness can be adjusted by adding more dates.

Green Tea Smoothie

1 packet of matcha green tea powder

1 to 3 pitted dates, depending on how sweet you would like it to be

1 teaspoon vanilla flavor or vanilla powder (optional)

1 cup nondairy milk or filtered water

½ banana (optional)

1 small handful of ice (optional)

Blend all ingredients together on high for a minute or two and then drink!

Matcha green tea is a great energy booster and substitute for coffee. It still contains caffeine, but it holds your energy at a steady level instead of giving you that sudden boost-and-drop you feel from coffee.

Maca Smoothie

1 tablespoon maca powder

1 frozen banana (you can peel and cut the banana into pieces and place them in the freezer the night before)

2 dates, pitted

1 teaspoon vanilla powder (optional)

1 teaspoon cinnamon

1 cup almond milk or soy milk

½ cup ice

Put all the ingredients into a blender. Blend on high for 2 minutes or until all ingredients are well blended together.

Maca is an adaptogen, which means that it helps regulate hormones and stress. Maca has been used to help regulate hormones during menopause and and to diminish other associated symptoms such as hot flashes. Not to mention it tastes like caramel.

Smoothie Bowl

Both frozen acaí or dragon (pittaya) fruit are great options, but any berries, fresh or frozen, will do.

LIQUID BASE
1 cup frozen acai or dragon fruit, or other frozen berries

2 cups filtered water or nondairy milk, such as almond, hemp, or soy milk

ADDITIONAL INGREDIENTS
2–3 pitted dates or 1 tablespoon maple syrup

½ to 1 banana

⅓ cup strawberries, fresh or frozen

1 tablespoon almond butter (optional)

handful of kale, cleaned, dried, and chopped after removing the stems

TOPPINGS
crushed walnuts, pecans
hemp seeds
goji berries
blueberries
blackberries
strawberries
sliced banana
mango
shredded coconut (raw or toasted)
pineapple
granola
mint leaves, sliced
cacao nibs
maple syrup (just a little drizzle)

Blend all of the ingredients together and pour into a bowl and arrange your toppings of choice to make a lovely presentation.

Topped Toast

1 slice of your favorite bread

¼ avocado, cut lengthwise into thin slices

2 slices tomato or small number of cherry tomatoes, chopped

dash of sea salt and pepper or favorite seasonings

Arrange avocado slices on the toast, top with tomato slices, then season with salt and pepper. You can shave a bit of lemon zest on top for a little tang.

OTHER GREAT TOPPINGS FOR TOAST
sautéed mushrooms and sautéed or caramelized onions

almond butter with banana and cinnamon

sliced apples and a sprinkle of cinnamon

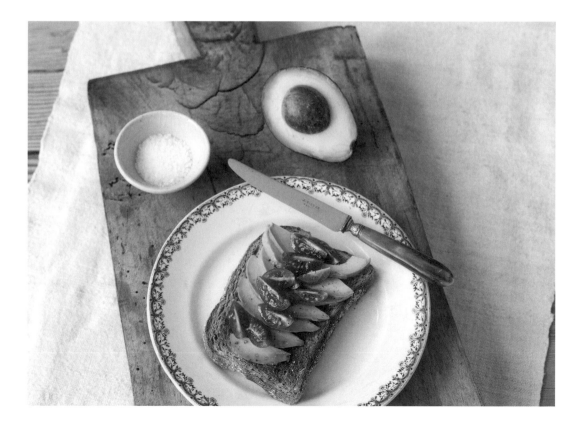

These meals can be served as lunch or dinner. Anything left over from dinner can easily be served as lunch for the following day. I even suggest having a salad or a nice vegetable soup for breakfast, as they are soothing and easy on the digestive system.

Salads

You can usually find prewashed salad greens and some prewashed vegetables, such as shredded carrots, in your grocery store. While they are a little bit more expensive than the unwashed produce, this is a nice time-saver. You will notice that I do not have salt listed in many of the recipes, or it's listed as optional. If you do want to add salt to any of the salad dressings, add a pinch of sea salt and black pepper to taste. Or see if you can go without it, and you will notice that after a while your taste buds will become more sensitive to the pure flavors of the food.

Kale Salad

dino kale, washed, drained, with stems removed

carrots, thinly sliced or grated

scallions (green part only), sliced

apple, seeds removed, then diced or chopped (Fuji apples are my favorite, and they work well in this recipe. Gala apples also work well.)

¼ avocado, cut into small pieces

¼ cup cilantro, washed, stems removed and chopped

DRESSING

1 teaspoon apple cider vinegar

1 teaspoon maple syrup or honey (if using coco aminos, you may want to leave out the honey or maple syrup)

¼ cup toasted sesame oil

1 teaspoon tamari or coco aminos

salt and ground black pepper to taste (optional)

Put all dressing ingredients into a glass jar. Close the lid and shake vigorously to mix. Or blend ingredients in a small blender.

Put the kale in a bowl. Then add the dressing and use your hands to massage the dressing into the kale. This allows the kale to soften a little bit. Let it sit for about 5 minutes. Then add the other ingredients and use a fork and spoon to incorporate them into the salad. Add more dressing if needed.

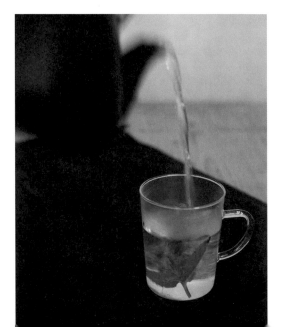

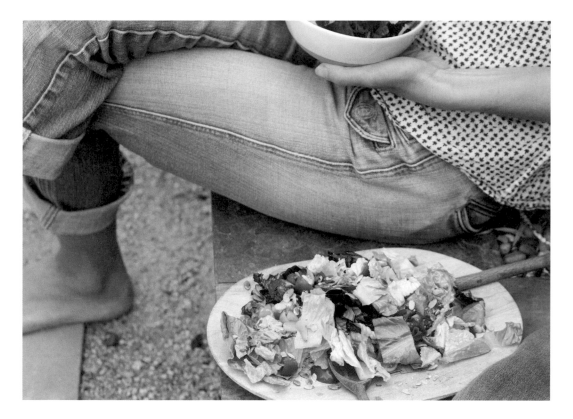

Romaine Salad

1 head of romaine lettuce (or the amount you want to use for your salad)

½ cup sliced red cabbage, either raw or sautéed

1 cup sautéed mushrooms (brown, button, maitake)

¼ cup pepitas, toasted

Wash and dry the lettuce.

Peel and discard the outer layer of leaves from the red cabbage. (You can slice the head in half and store one half for another time.) Thinly slice the amount you need.

With a damp paper towel, clean any dirt off the mushrooms.

Preheat a saucepan over medium heat.

Once the pan is hot, add 1/4 cup of water or just enough to get the bottom of the pan sizzling. This is water sautéing, and is a clean way to pan-cook vegetables without using oil.

Add the mushrooms and stir.

If the pan starts to get dry, add a little more water and continue to stir.

Season, if you wish, with pepper, any dry herbs like oregano or thyme, and a little sea salt (1/2 tsp). The mushrooms will readily absorb the salt.

Toast the pepitas over medium heat in a small pan. Watch them carefully, as they cook quickly. Once they are cooked, set them aside to cool.

Once all ingredients have cooled, place romaine, mushrooms, and cabbage in a bowl. Add the dressing and stir all ingredients together. Top with the pepitas, which will add a nice crunch to the dish.

DRESSING
¼ cup tahini

½ cup cilantro

½ cup parsley

juice of ½ lemon

2 cloves of garlic, minced

enough water to help thin the tahini

Put the ingredients in a blender and blend until smooth.

Cooking note: You can also experiment with adding other herbs, such as basil, dill, or tarragon. You can also add a raw red, yellow, or orange bell pepper, with seeds removed, into the dressing as well.

Butter Lettuce Salad

1 head butter lettuce

1 to 2 ears fresh white corn, or canned corn that has been rinsed. (When cutting the corn from the cob, be sure to be in control of your knife.)

1 vine ripened tomato, or a handful of cherry tomatoes either whole or sliced in half

¼ avocado cut into pieces

1 can black beans, rinsed and drained

CILANTRO DRESSING
1 bunch cilantro, stems removed

2 or 3 cloves garlic

1 teaspoon honey or maple syrup

1 teaspoon Dijon mustard

¼ cup olive oil

Blend all ingredients together in a blender. Then pour desired amount over salad and mix.

Soups

tip: When making soup, if you are using a store-bought stock or broth, make sure it's low in sodium so you have more control over the amount of sodium in the recipe.

Vegetable Soup

1 tablespoon olive oil or coconut oil

1 onion, halved and thinly sliced

5 cloves of garlic, minced or chopped

1 or 2 carrots, chopped

1 or 2 stalks celery, chopped

1 head broccolini, cut into bite-sized pieces

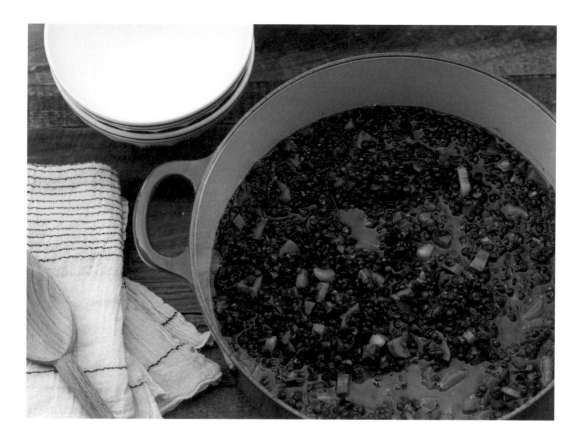

1 cup kale packed, stems removed, chopped

2 containers of low-sodium vegetable broth

juice of ½ lemon (approximately 1 tablespoon)

Place the pot on medium heat. Allow the pot to heat, then add the oil and make sure it is distributed all around the bottom of the pot. Add the onion and cook until translucent. Add the garlic and stir constantly so it doesn't burn.

Add the carrot and cook for about 8 minutes. Then add the celery and cook until it's translucent. Finally, add in the broccoli. Stir the ingredients together and add the vegetable broth or stock. Set the heat on high and allow the ingredients to come to a boil, then cover and simmer for 25 to 30 minutes. Add the kale for the last 5 minutes of cooking as well as a little bit of salt.

Feel free to add in any dry herbs you like, such as oregano, thyme, basil or bay leaves. Be sure to remove the bay leaves before serving.

Adjust the seasonings as needed. The lemon will help brighten up the flavors.

White Bean Soup

- 1 tablespoon extra virgin olive oil or coconut oil

- 1 teaspoon dried oregano

- 1 teaspoon fresh thyme (or simply add 3 sprigs to be removed at the end of cooking)

- 1 can cannelloni beans, rinsed and drained

- 1 large yellow onion

- 2 cloves garlic, chopped or minced

- 1 can diced tomatoes

- 2 containers low-sodium vegetable broth or stock

- 2 cups packed dino kale, washed, stemmed, chopped (feel free to try Swiss chard or bok choy instead of kale)

- juice of ½ lemon

Heat the oil in a pot over a medium flame.

Add the chopped onion and cook until translucent. Add the garlic and stir frequently so it doesn't burn. Add in the herbs.

Pour in the tomatoes and beans and stir.

Pour in the broth and bring to a boil. Then simmer on low heat for 30 minutes.

Add the kale for the last 5 minutes of cooking.

Season the soup with a little bit of sea salt and the lemon juice. Adjust the seasonings as needed.

Bowls

Bowls are a great way to have a variety of healthy ingredients in one dish. As you become more familiar with making bowls and with the possible ingredients, you can start getting more creative and experiment with your favorite seasonings, dressings, and vegetables to create new combinations.

As a base, use any whole grain, such as quinoa, brown rice, basmati rice, or millet. Use any of the salad dressings as a sauce.

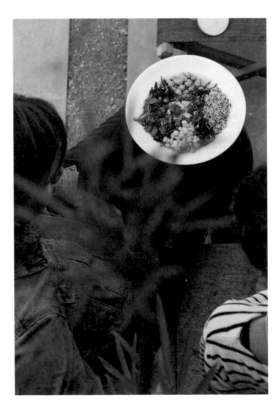

Quinoa Bowl

1 cup quinoa (or other whole grain)

½ cup white corn (fresh or canned corn, rinsed and drained)

½ cup tomatoes, chopped (vine ripened, heirloom, or cherry tomatoes cut in half)

½ cup carrot, shredded or grated

½ red onion, sautéed (optional)

½ red cabbage, sautéed

1 tablespoon pepitas, toasted

1 tablespoon fresh cilantro, chopped

If using quinoa, lightly toast it in a dry pan (no oil) for 5 minutes. Then boil two cups water and add the one cup of quinoa. Simmer on low, with lid, until the water has cooked out (about 10 minutes). Watch it to make sure the bottom doesn't burn.

Scoop the quinoa into a bowl.

Arrange the next 5 ingredients next to one another in the bowl. Have fun and experiment with the rainbow of colors possible with this dish!

Add the dressing of your choice

Sprinkle the pepitas and cilantro on top

Variation: As a substitute for the dressing, make a simple peanut sauce.

PEANUT SAUCE
¼ cup peanut butter or almond butter

1 tablespoon apple cider vinegar

1 tablespoon soy sauce or tamari.

HEAT
If you like spicy heat, add a jalapeño or serrano pepper. The heat will warm you up, and can help fire up your immune system as well.

tip: Add a little more flavor by cooking the quinoa in a vegetable stock or broth instead of water.

Warm Dishes

Baked Sweet Potato

1 sweet potato

¼ cup cooked black beans

¼ red, yellow, or orange bell pepper, chopped

Preheat oven to 425° F.

Wash the potato and dry it. Punch a few holes in the potato with a fork. Wrap it in foil and place on an aluminum foil or a parchment lined baking dish and place in the oven.

Bake for approximately 30 to 35 minutes or until potato is soft.

While the potato is cooking, sauté the bell pepper and set aside.

When the potato has finished cooking, add the cooked black beans to the dish. Top with the cilantro dressing or with guacamole.

Easy Vegetable Sauté

1 tablespoon coconut oil

1 yellow onion

2 cloves garlic

1 celery stalk

1 cup broccolini

1 carrot, shredded or chopped

½ bell pepper (any color), large dice

2 stalks of bok choy, cut into large pieces

1 tablespoon mint, chopped

¼ cup tamari or 3 tablespoons coco aminos

tip: If you use tamari, do not add any salt to the dish until after you have tasted it, since tamari is quite salty.

Place a saucepan over medium heat.

Add the oil and wait until it's hot.

Add the onion and cook until it begins to caramelize a bit.

Add the garlic, stirring constantly.

Add the celery and bell pepper.

Allow the ingredients to cook for 5 or 6 minutes.

Add the bok choy and carrot.

Cook until the bok choy just begins to wilt and turn bright green.

Turn off the stove and add the tamari or coco aminos and stir.

Add the fresh chopped mint as a garnish.

Eat this dish on its own or on top of rice or quinoa.

Whole Grain Pasta with Cannelloni Beans and Pesto

1 package whole grain pasta (follow cooking directions on package)

14 oz can cannelloni beans rinsed and drained

zest of 1 lemon

1 tomato, chopped, or ¼ cup whole cherry tomatoes (optional)

PESTO

1 cup packed basil

½ cup flat leaf parsley

½ cup mint

2 cloves garlic, chopped

⅓ cup walnuts, toasted

½ cup olive oil

juice of ½ lemon

½ teaspoon salt (optional)

½ teaspoon black pepper

While the pasta is cooking, begin to prepare the other ingredients.

Toast the walnuts in a saucepan over medium heat until they're just brown. Set aside to cool.

Place the basil, mint, parsley, garlic, olive oil, lemon, salt, and pepper and the cooled walnuts in a blender or food processor and blend together. Pour into a bowl and set aside.

Place the pasta in a large bowl. Add the pesto sauce along with the beans, and mix everything together. If you are adding tomatoes, add them at this step as well. Add the lemon zest and enjoy!

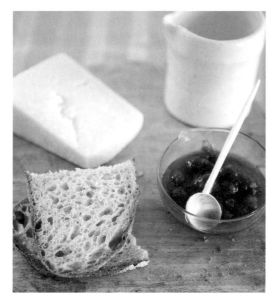

Snacks

Quick snacks could include:

Whole fruit or sliced fresh fruit—strawberries, mango, pineapple, melons, banana. You can also create any combination of fresh fruits to make a fruit salad.

Brown rice cakes or sesame crackers—brown rice cake spread with almond butter and topped with raspberries, sliced strawberries, apples, or banana, with a prinkle of cinnamon are one of my favorites.

Veggie sticks—cut up cucumbers and carrots, keep them in a glass of water with a squirt of lemon juice and leave them out to nosh on throughout the day.

Collard Wrap

Collard wraps make great snacks. You can substitute the collards for bread. Collard greens do have a thick stem. To prepare a leaf for a wrap, cut off the bottom stem. The spine is also very thick, so I take a knife and trim the spine to be about the same thickness as the leaf.

1 tablespoon hummus

sprouts

grated carrot

sliced avocado

tomato

cucumber

bell pepper

pesto

salad dressings

Choose any ingredients from the list above.

Spread hummus, pesto, or dressing on the collard leaf.

Then layer the other ingredients, as if you were making a burrito.

Roll the wrap and enjoy!

Stuffed Endives

Endives are versatile and make great bite-sized finger foods when filled with other ingredients.

STUFFINGS
hummus or baba ganoush

kalamata olives, chopped

dill, chopped

bell pepper, diced

carrot, diced or grated

cucumber

Cut the stem from the bottom of the endives.

Separate the leaves.

Spread hummus on a leaf, then add some olives and bell peppers.

Create different variations with the above ingredients.

Sweet Treats

Banana Ice Cream

4 frozen ripe bananas, cut into small pieces

For this recipe to be successful, you need ripe bananas. Ripe bananas have brown spots and are soft in texture.

Peel the bananas and cut them into small uniform pieces. Place them in a sealed zip lock bag, with all air removed. Let sit for 4 hours or overnight.

Remove the bananas from the freezer. I let mine sit out while I am setting up. You will need either a high-speed blender like a Vitamix or a food processor. I feel the food processor works best for this recipe.

Place the frozen bananas in the food processor. Blend until the banana becomes the consistency of soft serve ice cream. Scoop out and serve.

Top the banana with chopped pecans, almond or peanut butter, fresh strawberries, mint, or cacao nibs.

VARIATIONS
1 tablespoon peanut butter—add to the processor and blend with the banana

½ cup packed fresh mint (for mint chip ice cream, stir in fresh cacao nibs after removing banana and mint mixture from the processor)

1 tablespoon raw cacao powder and 1 table-spoon maple syrup or honey for a chocolate delight

½ cup blended strawberries—add them to the banana ice cream for a banana strawberry swirl

Fresh Fruit Topped with Pecan Cream

1 cup pecans, soaked overnight or for at least four hours in filtered water, then drained and rinsed

sweetener, such as maple syrup or honey, added slowly until desired sweetness is reached

1 teaspoon cinnamon

1 teaspoon vanilla flavoring

water

In a blender, combine the pecans, maple syrup or honey, cinnamon, and vanilla. Add a little bit of water, beginning with about a 1/4 cup. Begin blending on low speed and gradually increase to high. Add small amounts of water as needed in order to get a creamy consistency like whipping cream.

This goes really well on top of strawberries. You can add it to your oatmeal in the morning. Try also shaving some dark chocolate on top of the cream.

Variation: Cut a Fuji apple into thin slices, or cut the apple horizontally across into 3 layers; a top, a middle, and a bottom layer. On top of the slices or between the layers add the cream, raisins, a sprinkle of maca powder and cinnamon.

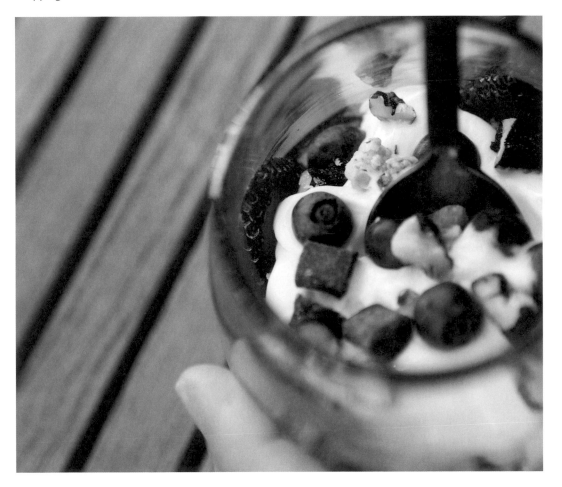

Richelle's Affirmations

Affirmations, some people cynically say, are lies you tell yourself until you believe them to be true. But at their simplest, they are a way of training your mind to produce positive, beneficial thoughts about yourself instead of negative ones.

I didn't enter the world of affirmations easily. I thought that the practice was silly and I didn't understand how saying these words to myself could possibly change my experience of life. I kind of got there through the back door. Louise L. Hay's book *You Can Heal Your Life* was my first foray into the world of affirmations. I had to pick it up and put it down a few times before any of it stuck.

But what the concept of affirmations did for me was to shine light on what I was already affirming, which was a lot of self-judgment and criticism, "what ifs," and readying myself for worst-case scenarios. It was not healthy or loving. Once I began to follow a funky feeling backward to where it originated, it always landed me in negative self-talk: thoughts in which I was claiming or saying something bad about myself or how something was going to go horribly wrong. I was so surprised. I was talking to myself in ways that I would never speak to another person, especially someone I loved. I would hear myself saying things like *You're not pretty enough, You're the wrong shape,* or *You'll never be picked, you're not smart enough.* One that I used on myself for years was *You're too late, you're too old!* I was never quite sure about what I was too late for, though: this started at age thirteen.

Here are some affirmations you can try

I put them up next to my bed so I see them before I sleep:
"Sleep comes easy, I wake restored."

I put them on my mirror:
"You are beautiful and easy to love."

I have one that comes up on my phone every day:
"Everything required is being accomplished in a relaxed and easy manner."

"I am perfect, powerful, and ready for an amazing life."

"My body is love, grace, ease, and abundant health."

"I am Inspired and In Spirit at all times."

So okay, I thought, if thinking these thoughts has me walking around feeling bad and crappy and sure that nothing is going to work out, maybe thinking good thoughts about myself will have the opposite effect.

I chose one affirmation and stuck with it, no matter how awkward it felt. I repeated it to myself, and also aloud, over the next several days. There was a shift in how I felt within just a few days. Sometimes in the very moment of speaking an affirmation out loud, I could feel myself open up or stand up a little taller. And then something very interesting happened. I began believing it. It was like a song that you just keep repeating the chorus to without being aware of it. Before I knew it, I was walking around more confident, lighter, and happier. Nothing notable in my external circumstances had changed to create the happiness I felt inside, but because I'd changed the way I spoke to myself, my interactions with people changed for the better. They became easier. I began to really look at who was in front of me. I affirmed that something was going to be easy, a conversation or an audition, and it was. If it was challenging, I remained easy within the challenge, which changed the outcome.

For example, I have affirmed that I am always right on time. I have used this more times than I can count and somehow everything lines up perfectly so that I am on time. And if I was late by the clock's time it has somehow worked out for the best. The real gift was not that I was paying more attention to time, but that I was more at ease in my body, my attitude, and the easy energy that surrounded me. When the judgments and negative thinking came up I replaced them with *I am joy and perfect in my own way; all is well.*

This is a process. Sometimes it will flow easily, and at other times there will be more resistance. Breathe and

Create a few of your own that speak to you

I am the perfect person for such a time as this.

I am the embodiment of the divine.

I am wealthy in all ways.

I am . . . (choose).

I know . . . (choose).

Now take a moment to choose or create one or two affirmations. Open your mind and heart to them every time you read them. Make them welcome.

continue. If there is resistance you've hit on something a little deeper, something that has a stronger root. That's a good thing. Breathe deeply and affirm you're good.

I have used affirmations in this way for almost forty years now. It's been a well-used tool.

I haven't been perfect at it; other thoughts still get in, of course. We are human. If you find yourself criticizing yourself or beating yourself up, be gentle and compassionate with yourself, and then choose another, more loving, thought for yourself. When I was moving into my mid to late fifties, I noticed my face and body changing and would often say to myself, *You look old*. This was completely unconscious. Once I'd caught myself, I realized I had been saying that to myself daily for several months whenever I looked in the mirror. Once I caught myself, I stopped immediately and created an affirmation. I began saying, *WOW, you're beautiful, and what a powerful body you have!*, every time I looked in the mirror. Not even a week later, my partner said to me, "Wow, you look beautiful. Have you started doing that Pilates CD? Your body looks really fit." I had already seen the shift.

It may seem corny at first, but it's a corny that really works!

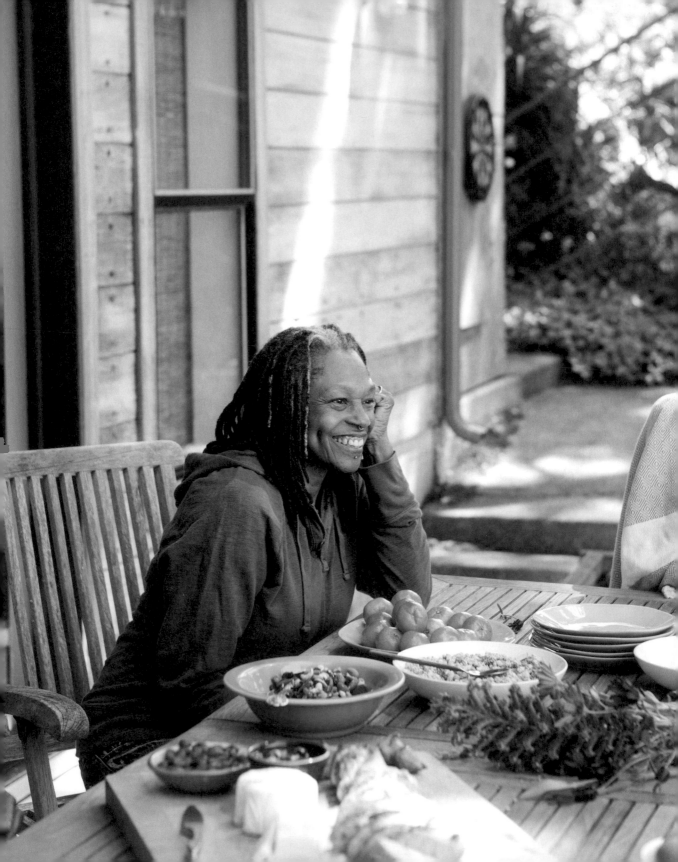

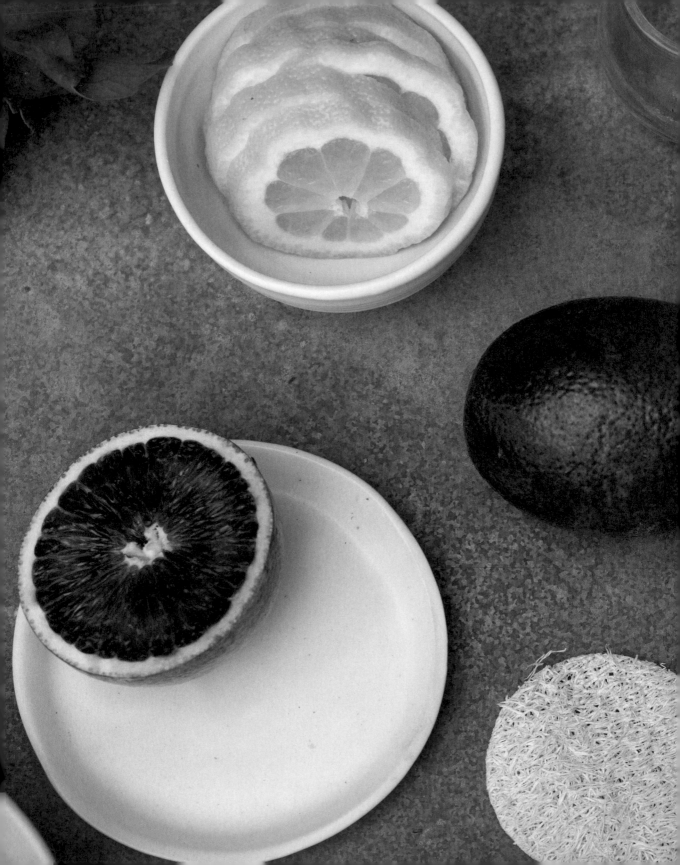

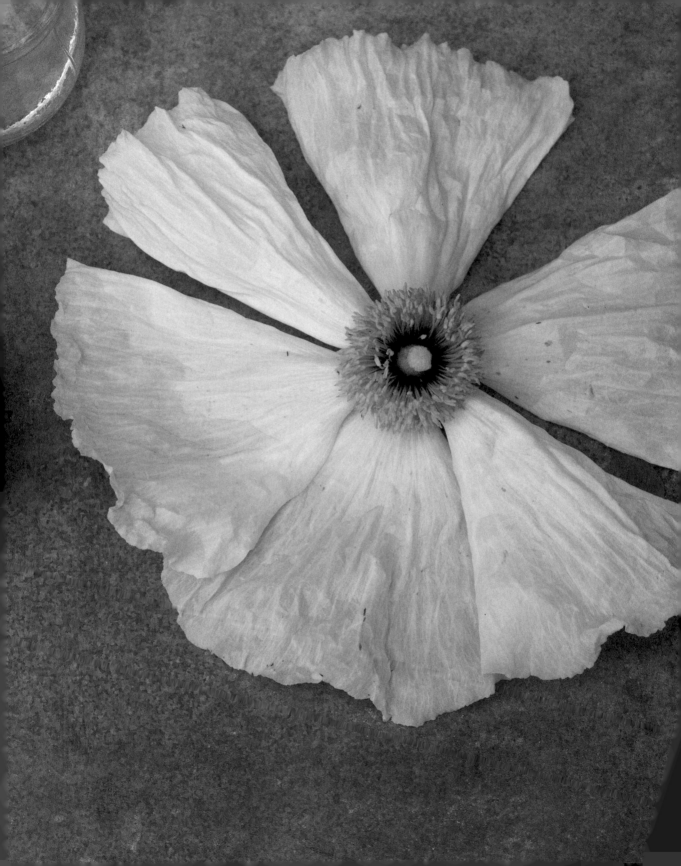

Playlists for a Long Weekend

Playlists are fun to make and can literally help you set the tone of your retreat. Upbeat, down-tempo, or flowing in between, the sound vibration of music can inspire you toward dancing, contemplation, sadness, and joy.

After the weekend is over, playing the songs can bring back sweet memories of your retreat and remind you of its atmosphere.

Richelle's Easy Grooves Playlist

— Gina Breedlove, "Breath"
— Indie Arie, "Strength, Courage and Wisdom"
— Sade, "Paradise"
— Toni Childs, "Walk and Talk Like the Angels"
— Bethovas Obas, "So Why?"
— Corrine Bailey Rae, "Butterfly"
— Gato Barbieri, "Europa (Earth's cry, Heaven's smile)"
— RUBY, "Listen O' Drop"
— Kerala Dream, "Jai Hanuman"

Rachel's Walk or Run in the Woods Playlist

— Calvin Harris, "Feels"
— Tribe Called Quest, "El Segundo"
— Pharcyde, "Passin Me By"
— Rhianna, We Found Love
— Shuggie Otis, "Outta My Head"
— Joan Armatrading, "Me, Myself, and I"
— Le Tigre, "After Dark"
— Beastie Boys, "No Sleep Till Brooklyn"
— Sky Ferreira,, "Everything is Embarassing"
— Ozomotli, "Stand Up Revolution"
— Khalid, "Location"
— Owl City, "Not All heroes Wear Capes"

Richelle's Dancin' Fools Playlist

_ Pharrell Williams, "Happy"
_ Jill Scott, "Living My Life Like It's Golden"
_ Prince, "Starfish and Coffee"
_ Earth Wind and Fire, "Fantasy"
_ Chaka Khan, "This Is My Night"
_ Beyonce, "Crazy in Love"
_ Ed Sheeran, "Barcelona"
_ Jamiroquai, "Seven Days in Sunny June"
_ Stevie Wonder, "Don't You Worry 'bout
   a Thing"
_ Micheal Franti, "What I Be"
_ Zap mama, "Bandy Bandy"
_ Rihanna, "Only Girl in the World"

Rachel's Cooking for One or a Whole Mess of People Playlist

_ Beyonce, "If I Were a Boy"
_ Josh Franklin, "Aint Nobody"
_ Sam Smith, "Too Good at Goodbyes"
_ Erykah Badu, "Phone Down"
_ Solange, "Rise"
_ Chance the Rapper, "No Problem"
_ Public Enemy, "Don't Believe the Hype"
_ Cutris Mayfield, "The Revolution Will Not
   Be Televised"
_ Common/De La Soul, "Getting Down in the
   Amphitheater".
_ Adele, "When We Were Young"
_ Alicia Keys, "Distance and Time"
_ Manau Chao, "Clandestino"

Grocery List for a Long Weekend

These are suggestions meant to spark inspiration. Buy the food that nourishes you and treats that genuinely make you feel good. Let your location, the season, your needs, and your group determine what you get. If you're having a long weekend with others, split up the list. Prioritize in-season and organic fruits and vegetables when available and affordable.

Fruits

_ Apple

_ Berries—strawberries, blackberries, and blueberries (if these aren't in season, usually you can find frozen versions that work well for smoothies and cereals)

_ Lemon

_ Lime

_ Pineapple

_ Orange

_ Grapefruit

_ Banana (fresh and / or frozen)

Vegetables

_ Avocado

_ Broccoli

_ Carrots (you can also purchase pre-grated carrots to save time)

_ Celery

_ Collard Greens

_ Cucumber

_ Cauliflower

_ Endive

_ Dino Kale

_ Mushrooms

_ Red Onion

_ Yellow Onion

_ Tomato

_ Romaine or Butter Lettuce

_ Red Cabbage

_ Garlic

_ Bell Pepper (red, yellow, orange)

_ Chile Peppers (jalapeño, serrano are good if you like spice)

_ White Corn

_ Swiss Chard

Herbs and Spices

_ Cilantro
_ Mint (fresh)
_ Oregano (dried and / or fresh)
_ Flat Leaf Parsley
_ Tarragon (fresh)
_ Thyme (fresh and / or dried)
_ Vanilla

Grains, Legumes, Beans, Oats

_ Brown Rice
_ Quinoa
_ Millet
_ Black Beans
_ Cannelloni Beans
_ Whole Grain Pasta
_ Oatmeal or Granola

Nuts, Seeds, Dried Fruit, Snacks

_ Walnuts
_ Pepitas (pumpkin seeds)
_ Chia Seeds
_ Almonds
_ Cashews
_ Goji Berries
_ Shredded Coconut
_ Dried apples or mango
_ Cocoa nibs to snack on

Oils, Vinegars, Condiments

_ Extra Virgin Olive Oil
_ Apple Cider Vinegar
_ Almond Butter
_ Dijon Mustard
_ Sesame Oil
_ Tahini
_ Tamari
_ Honey Maple Syrup
_ Celtic Sea Salt
_ Ground Black Pepper
_ Vegetable Broth (low sodium)
_ Hummus
_ Fresh Kalamata Olives

Dairy or Dairy Substitutes

_ Yogurt (Cow or Coconut)
_ Milk (Cow or almond, cashew, or soy)

Drinks

_ Seltzer or soda water
_ Black , rooibos, green, and or mint tea
_ Coffee or a root-based coffee substitute
   (Dandy Blend, Caffix, or Pero)

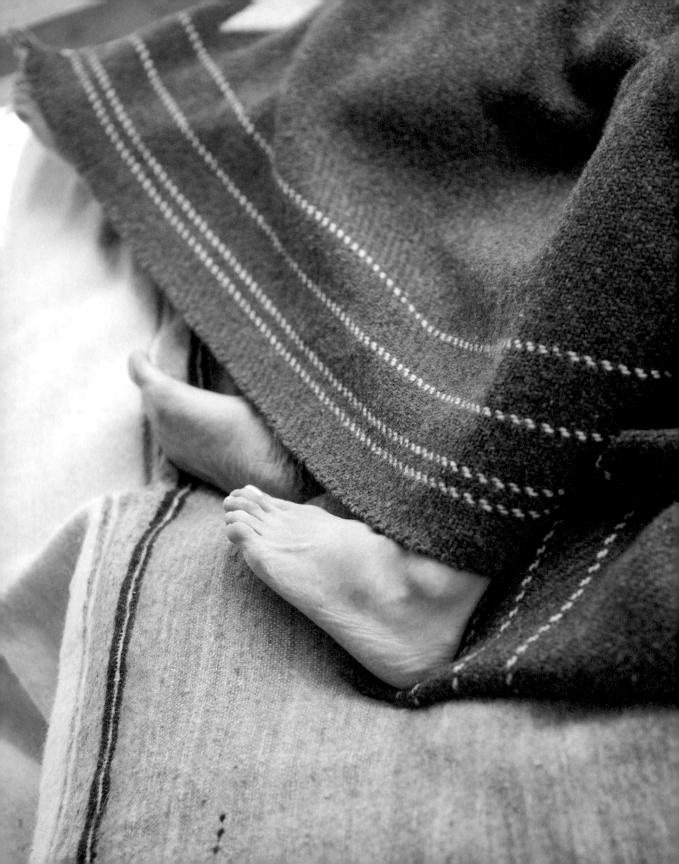

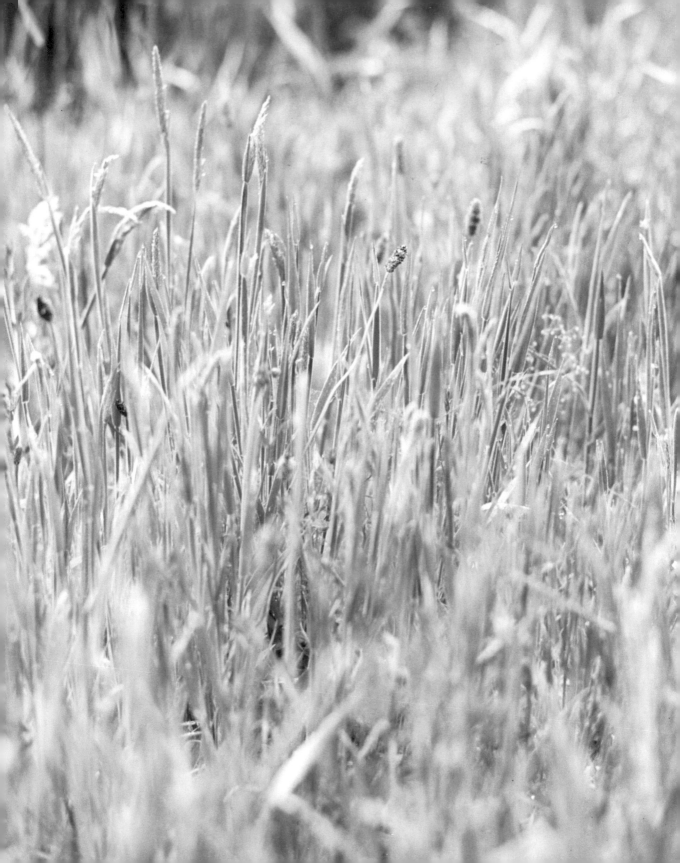

Retreat Centers

While you can plan your long weekend anywhere, if you'd like to go to a place designated for retreat, here are a few of the many worth checking out. All of the centers below are open to people of any cultural or spiritual backgrounds.

Plum Village
Plum Village has mindfulness practice centers in the tradition of Zen Master Thich Nhat Hanh in New York, Mississippi, California, and throughout the world.
plumvillage.org

Insight Meditation Center
Located in Barre, Massachusetts, IMS is one of the Western world's oldest Buddhist meditation retreat centers.
dharma.org

Kripalu
The Kripalu Center for Yoga and Health is a non-profit organization that operates a health and yoga retreat in Stockbridge, Massachusetts
kripalu.org

Esalen Institute
Nestled next to the Pacific Ocean, Esalen is a non-profit American retreat center and intentional community in Big Sur, California focusing on alternative education. Participants must register for a pre-organized retreat to attend.
esalen.org

Feathered Pipe Ranch
Feathered Pipe in Helena, Montana offers the ability to go on a personal retreat or scheduled retreats in a beautiful mountain setting.
featheredpipe.com

Ghost Ranch
Ghost Ranch is a gorgeous 21,000-acre retreat and education center in north central New Mexico. It is available for self-organized personal and group retreats of any length as well as participation in pre-organized events. Ghost Ranch is run by the Presbyterian Church and is open to the general public.
ghostranch.org

Shambhala Mountain Center

SMC is a non-profit Buddhist organization in northern Colorado whose mission is to create a space for the "exploration of individual and social wisdom."
shambhalamountain.org

Omega Institue

Omega is an educational retreat center in Rhinebeck, New York with workshops, natural food and beautiful surroundings. There are multiple classes available every day as well as workshops.
eomega.org

Venture Retreat Center

Venture is a non-denominational 22-acre retreat center just south of San Francisco, California. It is available for group and private retreats.
ventureretreat.org

Breitenbush Hot Springs Retreat

Breitenbush is a remote forest location with hot springs in Oregon. Personal and pre-organized retreats are available.
breitenbush.com

Acknowledgments

Thank you to the beautiful people who modeled for us, cooked with us, played games with us, tried out new recipes and strange poses, and who make any moment a bit of a long weekend with their grace, humor, and love:

Gina Breedlove, Tali Sedgwick, Ai Kubo, Kelly Foster, Beth Protass, Carolyn Kelly, Kymi Armour, Nicki Clark, Ai Kubo Chrissy Mazzeo, Tali Sedgwick Waldman, Tanea Lynx, Yeshi Neumann, Beth Miles, Gina Spigarelli, and Sam Melendez. Thank you to the good people of Muir Beach, Bolinas, and Pachamama, Todos Santos for hosting our primary photoshoots.

In honor and loving memory of Yulanda "Chef" Hendrix.

About the Authors

Richelle Donigan is a Yoga Instructor, Life Mastery Coach and Consultant, and Inspirational Speaker. Through her teaching, speaking, and retreats, Richelle seeks to diversify all communities, creating inclusive practice spaces to make available and facilitate healing and well-being for all. Richelle has been featured in two films, *Warrior Marks* with Alice Walker and *Planet Yoga*. She has taught and facilitated retreats and workshops in the US, India, Mexico, Panama, and the UK. longweekendretreat.com

Rachel Neumann has led group creativity, grieving, yoga, mindfulness, and business retreats. Her stories have appeared in the *New York Times, AlterNet, The Village Voice,* and other publications. A Rockwood Leadership Institute Arts and Social Justice Fellow, Rachel's work was selected for the *Best Buddhist Writing 2013* anthology. rachelbneumann.com

About the Photographer

Ericka McConnell is a bicoastal Californian who has worked in New York for more than twenty years and has photographed retreat centers in India and Mexico, and in Santa Barbara and Santa Fe in the US. Her images have graced the covers of *Travel + Leisure, Woman Magazine, Fitness,* and *Yoga Journal.* Instagram @Erickamccfoto

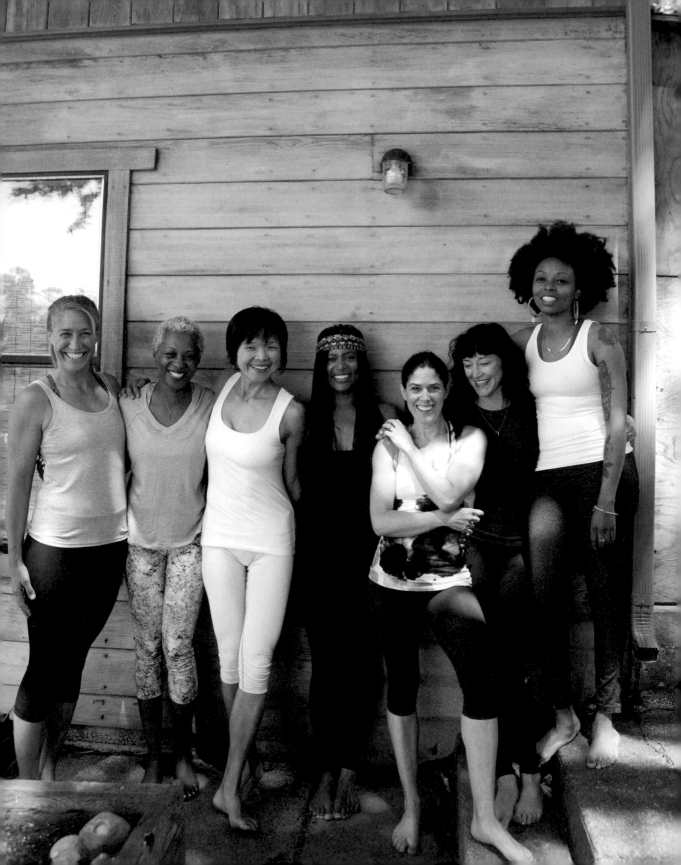

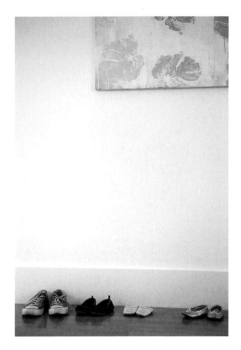

longweekendretreat.com

Parallax Press
P.O. Box 7355
Berkeley, CA 94707
parallax.org

Parallax Press is the publishing division of
Plum Village Community of Engaged Buddhism, Inc.
© 2018, Richelle Donigan and Rachel Neumann
Photography © Ericka McConnell
All rights reserved

Printed in Canada

Cover and text design by Debbie Berne
Richelle's author photograph © Bethany Hines
Rachel's author photograph © Jason DeAntonis

DISCLAIMER: The advice in this book is intended for general information purposes only. Any application of the material set forth in the following pages is at the reader's discretion and is their sole responsibility.

ISBN: 978-1-946764-02-7

Library of Congress Cataloging-in-Publication Data is available on request.

1 2 3 4 5 / 22 21 20 19 18

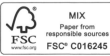

MIX
Paper from
responsible sources
FSC® C016245
FSC
www.fsc.org

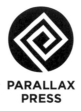

**PARALLAX
PRESS**

Parallax Press is a nonprofit publisher, founded and inspired by Zen
Master Thich Nhat Hanh. We publish books on mindfulness in
daily life and are committed to making these teachings accessible
to everyone and preserving them for future generations. We
do this work to alleviate suffering and contribute to a more just
and joyful world. For a copy of the catalog, please contact:

Parallax Press
P.O. Box 7355
Berkeley, CA 94707
parallax.org

31901062625324